MENOPAUSE
IS
HOT

Everything
You Need to
Know to Thrive

MARIELLA FROSTRUP
and ALICE SMELLIE

Foreword by NAOMI WATTS

SCRIBNER

New York Amsterdam/Antwerp London Toronto Sydney New Delhi

Scribner
An Imprint of Simon & Schuster, LLC
1230 Avenue of the Americas
New York, NY 10020

Copyright © 2021 by Mariella Frostup and Alice Smellie
Originally published in Great Britain in 2021 by Bluebird,
an imprint of Pan Macmillan, as *Cracking the Menopause*

First Scribner hardcover edition January 2025

For information about special discounts for bulk purchases, please contact Simon & Schuster Special Sales at 1-866-506-1949 or business@simonandschuster.com.

The Simon & Schuster Speakers Bureau can bring authors to your live event. For more information or to book an event, contact the Simon & Schuster Speakers Bureau at 1-866-248-3049 or visit our website at www.simonspeakers.com.

Manufactured in the United States of America

1   3   5   7   9   10   8   6   4   2

Library of Congress Cataloging-in-Publication Data has been applied for.

ISBN 978-1-6680-6897-7
ISBN 978-1-6680-6896-0 (ebook)

To our mothers who made us think,
to our sisters and friends who made us talk,
and to our daughters who made us want to change their world.

Contents

MENOPAUSE IS HOT

Foreword

It gives me great pleasure to write a foreword to this surprising and important book about menopause, which is packed with biological facts and scientific research, and also with humor, warmth, and a sense of camaraderie: exactly how we need to approach this time of life. I've known Mariella for many years, and I am pleased that she is bringing her passion and drive for menopausal justice to the United States, both with the advocacy group Menopause Mandate US, which we co-chair, and with this vital book, which I hope will speak to American women of all ages who want to wise up about the menopausal transition.

When I was told I might be close to menopause at the age of thirty-six, there was very little information or even conversation about the topic, and the whole experience was riddled with shame and confusion. Had there been more resources, my menopausal transition over a decade ago would have been much easier. Nowadays, I am even more determined to raise awareness and make sure there is a community and a place for information to bring a sense of humanity to all of this.

Many women struggle in isolation, like I did, without the proper information needed to navigate the difficult times that this stage of life can bring. My menopause journey was long, confusing, and lonely on occasion. But I've come out the other side feeling stronger, more confident in my own skin, and more myself. Half the population goes through menopause, so we all deserve to know what's happening to our bodies and what we can do about it.

Incredibly, there is still shame around the subject. Shame about our bodies is so deeply ingrained in women. It starts as early as our periods: have we got them, are we bleeding too heavily, does it smell right . . . ? We then meet more culturally shameful waypoints through our lives. Carrying that shame with us, for years, is exhausting. But now the ice has finally been broken with menopause and women are far freer around the subject. It's almost like our version of war stories, "Let me tell you my scary story!" "Hear mine, it's even worse!" That ability to open up only comes with years and years of experience.

Thankfully, there's now a groundswell of information. Women are raising their hands and feeling safer about sharing their stories. This conversation— alongside education and research—is beginning to evolve. We've realized that menopause isn't simply about the end of our fertility, it's also about midlife. Since we're living so much longer, we need to optimize our health in every way. That includes our mental health and how we relate to our part- ners, our children, and the workplace.

As the conversations grow, people are more invested than ever in tak- ing care of themselves. I see the tides turning, and it's not just for women. Men are talking about it, too. Is menopause becoming cool, like a badge of honor? I hope so.

We need to remember that there is no one-size-fits-all solution. Each woman's experiences, symptoms, reactions, and body are different, and ev- eryone deserves to feel the best they can. Women need to know exactly how good and, for the most part, how safe menopausal hormone therapy (MHT) is. I know that some people don't want to take it, or it's not con- sidered safe for them, and that's fine; it's a personal decision to be made with your doctor. All I can say is, though I'm not a medical expert, it's been a game changer in my life. I went on MHT very early and have been on it for more than ten years with great results. Among other things, it's helped with my sleep. And if I can't sleep, I can't function or do anything else in my life, which leads to other problems: brain fog, anxiety, lack of confidence, mood swings . . . you name it. And then I won't be able to perform well as a mother or at my job. For me, MHT is vital.

It's interesting to go through something as personal as menopause while under public scrutiny, which comes with my line of work. I used to be called up to play the girl next door, damsel in distress, femme fatale, woman on the verge. Now it's woman in full-blown menopause, in her power. I'm trying to embrace my age—I think it only leads to better work. No one's calling on me anymore to play a twenty-five-year-old who's falling in love for the first time. I'm going to play a woman who's faced challenges and seen the other side of them. I've experienced grief, I've experienced loss, divorce, teenagers . . . and that informs every story I tell and every character I play. So why not lean into it, especially since trying to run from it is a fruitless endeavor?

There's a kind of peace that comes with being on the other side of menopause. Knowing that the symptoms will calm down, and the acceptance and tolerance of your physical and mental health is a real positive. You know what you like, and what you don't. With that knowledge comes confidence and control over yourself again. And that can be really powerful.

The unhealthy competition that can exist with other women dissipates, too. "Have you done this yet? Have you done that? What have you achieved? How many boxes have you ticked . . . ?" Now, if you haven't gotten to tick all the boxes, I think you've come to a place of ease. We can calm down and find a little bit of peace.

There's also a chance to reinvent yourself at this point in life. It's daunting, but it's doable. And we must be open to change; nests are emptying, kids are moving away, parents are aging. All things are shifting around you, and accepting that is a good thing.

My wish now is that our generation can end the silence and create a world where menopause is not a thing to be feared. As Mariella reminds us, it's by no means the end! We've taken the first steps, but there's still a long way to go. That's why a book like this is such a necessary read. We are so much stronger when armed with knowledge, and there's no force more powerful than women (and men) working together to change the world for the better.

Naomi Watts

Introduction

I know I speak for many women when I say that if menopause were a place you could visit, it wouldn't be a popular destination. Perhaps it would be an ancient gas station, set in the middle of a barren and rocky desert, with heavy gray skies and a battered wooden sign reading "Next Stop: Death." No wonder most of us still arrive at this pit stop in a state of terrible trepidation.

But there's a menopause revolution starting. The once forbidden topic of women's aging and changing biology is being embraced and discussed by luminaries from Michelle Obama to Oprah to Maria Shriver to Naomi Watts and Drew Barrymore, not to mention a host of brilliant doctors and campaigners like Dr. Sharon Malone and Dr. Mary Claire Haver. After millennia of misunderstanding, the diminishing of our fertility hormones is getting a rebrand; not as the devastating blow of outdated folklore, but as a new and exciting start, a second spring if you will. This turbulent season of change in midlife, a bit like puberty with wrinkles, is at last being understood as a liberation, rather than the agent of our redundancy. Our middle years now hold actual enticements, as a period of renewal and risk-taking, a time to fulfill unrealized ambitions and abandon unhealthy habits in our lives and relationships rather than fade quietly into an invisible old age.

With around two million women becoming menopausal every year in the US, and one in four women over the age of forty (around 83 million in total), there's certainly incentive to pick up the baton and keep running with it, rather than accepting the misogynistic view that after menopause women's currency goes into free fall. Tell that to the hordes of supremely successful women in midlife. To be clear, when we say "menopause" we're mostly using it as a blanket word, encompassing peri- to post- (which is generally your early forties till the end of your life)!

Just five years ago, had you told me that a word previously whispered in dark corners would become a global discussion, a badge of female honor, and something to be shouted from the rooftops, I'd have laughed with derision. Back then, I had only just finished a BBC documentary called *The Truth About the Menopause*. It had taken years to come to fruition, as I tried to understand why this compulsory life stage for all women was so shrouded in secrecy.

The documentary sparked huge interest in the UK; women began materializing in the strangest places—restaurant restrooms, grocery store aisles, at coffee shops and on sidewalks, thanking me for having the "courage" to say the unsayable. To my amusement, at a party in London, chatting to the handsome actor Michael Fassbender, I watched as he was pushed unceremoniously aside by a woman in her thirties who wanted to enthuse about my use of the M-word, leaving me to explain to Michael why menopause matters so much! I wonder if he's recovered.

That's when I realized that menopause was no laughing matter. With the floodgates prised open, it became apparent that this transition, experienced by half the global population, was woefully misunderstood, criminally ignored, and, like all matters of female health, desperately underfunded. It certainly ranked among the top five of patriarchal fails, no mean feat in a list that includes the gender pay gap, uneven division of domestic labor, and women and children being the primary victims of every war fought.

Women around the world are questioning why they are frequently being forced to resort to an unreliable internet to find out what's happening to their bodies in midlife. Read any menopause account on social media and the comments will constitute a list of women's firsthand testimonies: being dismissed by their doctors, suffering debilitating symptoms for years, and most shocking of all, denied hormone replacement therapy (HRT), also, and more recently known, as hormone therapy—HT or menopausal hormone therapy (MHT)—because you aren't "replacing" what's not there, point out more medically qualified minds than mine. MHT is what we've gone with in this book. There is still a lack of clarity over the safety of MHT, despite it being recognized as the best support for those going through the transition, which will be explained—in our MHT chapter we expose the flawed study that led to a global panic. For now, suffice it to say that although menopause experts globally are firmly in favor of MHT, there remains a cornucopia of hocus-pocus out there; with differing opinions, solutions, and diagnoses offered from state to state and doctor to doctor.

Until my late forties I'd believed myself to be a reasonably well-informed woman of the world, a journalist with three decades of campaigning on women's issues under my belt. *Then wham!* My ignorance about menopause knocked any such certainties firmly aside. I felt as though I was being sucked into a black hole, with no bearings and no idea of how to change course. The lack of clear direction around the transition is quite staggering, although with a map and rudimentary navigational tools it can be a relatively easy journey. But I, like so many of us, found myself stumbling solo through a maze of misinformation and confusion, without so much as a compass to point me in the right direction.

We need to drag the topic of menopause out of its dark corner and place it firmly in public discourse. It was a chat I'd never had—not with my mother, my friends, or even my doctor. When I was sixteen and living in Catholic Ireland, my mother helped me acquire birth control pills. She and I had talked about sex and death, divorce and bad periods, we'd battled her cervical cancer together and discussed the meaning of life when she was diagnosed with dementia, but we'd never, ever, ever talked about menopause. My only recollection of her mentioning this transitory period of her life was a fleeting comment in my late twenties about a hormone patch she had been given. This, she said, made her feel like an unmilked dairy cow—bloated and uncomfortable—a sliver of information that served to instill further foreboding. Nothing to look forward to there! Even in our most vocal of households, that was the closest we ever got to discussing this compulsory progression in every woman's biological journey.

Having left school in my midteens, I initially assumed that I'd simply missed, or skipped, the relevant biology class. But that lesson had never taken place. We all knew the word (and feared it), had a vague start date in our minds, and had heard of hot flashes. Other than that, what was increasingly apparent was that most women's knowledge about menopause could be jotted on one of my mother's short-lived MHT patches.

When I started to experience symptoms at the age of forty-nine, I had no idea what was happening. After all, I'd never been told that anxiety and insomnia were two of the most corrosive side effects of hormonal free fall. For two years I barely slept, raged at my husband and kids, and was swamped by levels of anxiety that were as debilitating as they were irrational. I don't think I've ever felt so alone. On the rare occasions when I mentioned my concerns to girlfriends ("I slept four hours last night, is this normal?"), they all seemed to have more questions than answers.

Sadly, this is the unfortunate experience for millions of women. We all know loosely what "menopause" means but we are ignorant of specifics—and, most importantly, that the ever-increasing list of symptoms can start up to ten years before, during what's known as perimenopause, and these are just as significant as the final closing of the curtains of our fertility.

What a strange anomaly this is. We're not thirteen-year-old girls confused by our changing bodies. Many of us are intelligent professionals who manage our finances, understand world affairs, and know how to put air into car tires, but are as perplexed as any teen in a training bra when it comes to details about this compulsory date in our fertility calendar.

What's more, we've been encouraged to believe that we're but a step away from our endgame, rather than—as I now firmly believe—on the brink of the second phase of our lives. Or, as esteemed OB/GYN Dr. Sharon Malone has described it, entering our "third trimester of life," years we believe are filled with possibility, adventure, and new, exciting relationships and career opportunities.

Like so many women I felt utterly defeated by the oppressive proximity of an inevitable future of dried-up sexual organs, hot flashes, lack of desirability, general shriveling, and ultimately loss of brain power and death. Psychologists warn against fight-or-flight mode, yet I found myself trapped in an unwinnable conflict with my own hormones, and feeling myself metaphorically diminishing and withering into the crone that society believed me to be.

In the hilarious sketch "Last F**kable Day," comedian Amy Schumer sharply illustrates how aging renders menopausal women undesirable overnight. Certainly, with symptoms like insomnia and anxiety taking their toll, desirability certainly wasn't in my top ten of worries. "Brazen Husky," as the UK newspaper the *Daily Mail* once summed up my charms, was certainly not what the world was seeing now! Clawing around for helpful information merely confirmed that the end of life as I'd previously known it was beckoning.

Eventually, at age fifty-one, a mere shadow of my former self, I went to see my OB/GYN in London, Sara Matthews. I've raved for years about her Jessica Rabbit–like elegance and tumbling Titian locks. But more important than her glamour—though I yearned for glamour as I was feeling so utterly drab—was the feeling of coming home as I sat down in her office and described how I felt. "We can't have you feeling like that," she said comfortingly, in her lovely Irish brogue. Not only did she hear me, but she immediately identified the problem. I was, without question, perimenopausal.

Once I realized that I was experiencing the menopausal transition, I felt as though I'd stumbled on the world's best-kept secret. What became rapidly evident was that, as with "natural birth," managing the symptoms of menopause by gritting your teeth and getting on with it (and definitely not discussing it in public) seemed to have become the litmus test for admirable stoic femininity. So I started to ask questions.

If menopause was barely mentioned among women, it was positively banned in the company of men. The only acceptable references were lewd comments in sleep-inducing stand-up comedian monologues and tepid sitcoms, where menopause and mother-in-law jokes have provided easy targets since time immemorial. "Why is menopause called menopause? Because mad cow disease was taken" is a prime example. Laugh? I think not. Making women feel marginalized and humiliated is no longer palatable or acceptable. As the slogan goes, "Time's up" on this, too.

Despite making up fifty percent of the global population, and without whom our species would perish, we were deemed an "invisible minority." Could things really be this cataclysmic? In 2018, when I set out to find answers with that BBC documentary, we barely scratched the surface of this topic, as television tends to do. It seemed a half-hour look into the science on mainstream TV was as much as women could expect, but I was overwhelmed with the tsunami of gratitude—and ratings to match.

Most of the time I felt utterly astonished at having done so little to provoke such a great response. Rather than feeling pride in my supposedly pioneering exposé, I felt even angrier that this phase in our lives, something so mundane and inevitable, should be the wellspring of so much shame, anxiety, ignorance, and fear. Once the conversation was started, and we were talking, it appeared that everyone wanted in on the discussion and women had a lot to say.

In addition to working as a radio and television journalist, I was an advice columnist for a major UK newspaper for two decades. This book is, in some ways, an extended (very extended!) advice column. Although narrated in my voice, it is very much a joint effort.

Back in 2020, Alice Smellie, my co-author and a health journalist, and I attended a menopause seminar at a five-star hotel deep in the English countryside. We watched a series of intelligent and articulate women display the same state of ignorance, saying that they were just going to "push on through." There was no thought of asking for support. That was the night we decided to write the book.

At the time, Alice and I had just started a running group with school mums. Everyone was ten years younger than me—I was a very late mother, having had both my children in my early forties. I found myself going on about my own perimenopause and then gradually the others caught up, and the outrage and symptom-discussing kept us going through many a 5K. Alice credits these intense discussions with her having experienced what she describes as the "shortest menopause ever"; flanked by myself and a friend who is a menopause nurse, her "anxiety" was instantly diagnosed as perimenopause and she was on MHT within the month.

I think of it as a staging post rather than a final destination, especially now, aged sixty-one, having traveled many more miles. But our culture still says otherwise. Puberty and pregnancy are seen as positive progressions, but menopause is when forward momentum halts and, like Shakespeare's "golden lads and girls," we begin to "come to dust." Men mature, while us dusty women wither, shrivel, and disintegrate.

In some ways, it's understandable that menopause should be deemed such a traumatic rite of passage. Our fertility is so deeply embedded in our psyches that, for many women, it feels like our raison d'être.

Suffering setbacks in pursuit of procreation or choosing to eschew it altogether can feel like a bereavement or a failure, as many women who've struggled with infertility, not met the right partner, or decided not to have children may have found. We've been told for millennia that our only point is to make babies, and we're made to feel it leaves a big gap on our résumé if we won't, haven't, or can't. As a result, menopause has culturally come to render women redundant, unlike any middle-aged man in the prime of his life.

Since a version of this book was published in the UK in 2021, I have spoken and written widely about menopause. Alongside politicians, celebrities, and journalists, I co-founded the campaign group Menopause Mandate, now in the US as well, which has at its heart a passion to educate and support women going through the menopausal transition.

With issues of women's health, wealth, rights, and happiness on the menu as never before, it's high time we dragged this third stage of our biological cycle out of the depths of Pandora's Box. Despite homo sapiens spending over 300,000 years on this planet, menopause appears to have been less explored than our oceans' deepest depths in the Mariana Trench: misdiagnosed, misappropriated, and misunderstood in a narrative composed almost entirely by men. Half the world's population is affected, but it remains one of the most toxic words in our lexicon, signaling the end of a woman's worth and value, the loss of libido, the general desiccating of organs, and the fast track to decline and death. With our increasing lifespans, we're often living over a third of our lives postmenopausal, leaving us with a generous and exciting new phase of existence. Women are beginning to realize that we've been far too silent about our biology and that it's not unreasonable for fifty percent of the global population to expect the way their bodies work to be respected and supported, rather than treated as a toxic shame to be swept under the carpet.

In chapter one, we'll take a whirlwind tour through the mostly pitiful, ignorant, and certainly highly biased "information" that has swirled around us for the last few thousand years. Chapter two onwards will take you through all things menopause in the modern age, with contributions from women with many different experiences. It's time to drag menopause and all the surrounding symptoms and experiences out into the sunlight. Only by joining the conversation, by airing and sharing, listening and learning will we progress from the position of ignorance to which we've been relegated for so long.

CHAPTER ONE

Pointless and Poisonous: Menopause in the First Millennia

Where do you start when you have centuries of ignorant assumptions and ludicrous diagnoses to condense into a few historical snapshots? Happily, we don't have to plunge back into the primordial swamps, as there isn't much reference to older women's bodies until the seventeenth century. Menopause is very much a medical afterthought, from classical times onwards. Being unique to women, it was obviously unimportant and uninteresting unless it impacted the lives of the ruling classes, who were, almost to a man, men. Looking back through the arch of history, you certainly come to the conclusion that menopause needs a spin doctor. As recently as 1969, the American doctor David Reuben, in his bestseller *Everything You Always Wanted to Know About Sex*, informs us that "As estrogen is shut off a woman becomes as close as she can to being a man." He continues: "Having outlived their ovaries, they may have outlived their usefulness as human beings."

This tone is common throughout the ages. There's a "Whoops, it's all over, love" subtext to almost every written word or comment made about the end of female fertility, whether it be medical or literary. Peering back to the first dim documentation certainly compounds the sense of looming disaster. If periods were called The Curse, then what followed was nothing short of a death sentence! Let's start with ancient times—those wonderful Greek and Roman men who were eternally immortalized in marble and are still studied by classics students. It's unlikely you'll be able to conjure up any female names unless they were goddesses.

Unsurprisingly, menopause wasn't prominent in the medical research or philosophical theories. Greek philosopher and revered thinker Aristotle managed one nearly accurate bit of detail around 300 BC, saying the average age at which fertility ceased was around forty, but it definitely happened by fifty. In fact, fifty-one is still widely quoted as being the average age at which we have our final period.

There was certainly no interest expressed about perimenopause, the years preceding menopause itself, when hormones start to go up and down like an opinion poll about the top ten hottest Greek gods. I'd be tempted to scrutinize Aristotle's pioneering philosophies with a stern eye if they are anything like his flawed description of women's bodies. According to him, women contain too much blood due to our coldness, general ineptitude, and less active lifestyle. (I wonder if he'd ever mopped the kitchen floor?) For the revered thinker, periods are the process of getting rid of the excess blood, and as we age we get drier, so periods stop, whereas men are constructed with perfect balance and just the right amount of heat and blood (which they make into semen). This idea of menstruation as a cleansing process of some sort endures for almost another two thousand years.

David Reuben was toward the end of a long line of such "experts" to offer the opinion that, as women go beyond menopause and their periods stop, they become more masculine, though, as he adds, "Not really a man, but no longer a functional woman." In some societies, including Ancient Greece, there were (and still are) freedoms given to postmenopausal women as they edge closer to the idealized marvelousness of men.

As we move on through the centuries, interest in menopause remains pretty static, a disinterested medical shrug. A sixth-century physician, Aetius of Amida, suggested that the "very fat cease early" (untrue, as it happens), and the "first female gynecologist," Trota of Salerno, was a voice of reason around the twelfth century in Italy. It's said that she wrote a major work on women's medicine in medieval Europe, *The Trotula*. Or did she? Did she exist? Was she in fact a man? This point was debated for centuries until academics cut through the historical haze to confirm her sex. I am pretty sure that, had she been a man, there'd be clear documentation and a large medical school named after him, with a big statue outside. The Father of Gynecology, he'd be called. Instead, the debate was: "We're unsure. Was Trotula a woman or a book?"

Then there's Saint Hildegard of Bingen in twelfth-century Germany, who was marvelously pioneering for the time. Her observation, "The menses cease in women from the fiftieth year and sometimes in certain ones from the sixtieth when the uterus begins to be enfolded and to contract so they are no longer able to conceive," may not be entirely accurate, but scarily it's not that far removed from our level of understanding today.

Hildegard, who founded two abbeys and wrote classical music that is still played today, very much flew the flag for postmenopausal success. Aged sixty, she went on four preaching tours, in spite of women having been forbidden to do so. And she was a member of the female sex, with hands-on experience, rather than one of the numerous mumbling men who felt qualified to offer their unqualified opinions on all matters female over the centuries.

Moving on up through our bloody—literally—history, in the Middle Ages our inability to get rid of what was now considered toxic blood meant that menopausal women were seen as bubbling cauldrons of poisons. We didn't have the strength to expel them, and suffered terribly, until we dropped dead from one of the many venoms we harbored. A little Aristotle clearly goes a long way when it comes to handing down "wisdoms."

The thirteenth-century German philosopher and scientist Albertus Magnus, whose day job was "German Catholic Dominican Bishop," was long credited with writing a dark tome called *De Secretis Mulierum* (Women's Secrets). This cheery book was filled with insights such as "The retention of menses engenders many evil humors." The author—and I think it's fair to suggest that he wasn't exactly a jolly family man—also believed that older women were poisonous and dangerous, with the ability to kill children just by looking at them. The latter is a skill that sometimes, when a teen is being particularly infuriating, would be a useful threat. "Be home by midnight, or I'll come in and LOOK at you."

What a typical menopausal reference though. The moment it's in any way interesting to medics, academics, and men—same thing—it's judged to be a scourge rather than a liberation. Any lack of credibility didn't hinder his career progress. Magnus was later canonized as Saint Albert the Great, patron saint of the natural sciences, and he is also credited with discovering arsenic. A life well led.

The sixteenth-century Italian doctor Giovanni Marinello, in *Le medicine partenenti alle infermità delle donne*, which roughly translates as "Medicine for Women's Problems" (1563), gives a less witchy, more medical, but nonetheless dismal description of any woman whose periods have halted. "Those women [ladies, that's you] . . . are always infirm and most of all in those parts of the body which are connected to and have some kind of correspondence with the uterus . . . thus as soon as the periods stop, pains arise, apostemata, eye disorders, weak sight, vomiting, fever; and they desire the male more than ever."

Ah, yes. You'll notice the mention of us desiring men. Another repulsive trait of menopausal women through the ages is our desperation for sex. During our fecund (fuckable) days, such interest in the male of the species might possibly be something to celebrate, but not when it's a menopausal hag doing the lusting.

Marinello continues for quite some time in the same vein: "The disorderly uterus rises or descends all the time or commits other actions difficult to endure. From this soon a tightness of the chest arises, faintings of the heart, breathlessness, hiccups, and other troublesome accidents, from which the woman sometimes dies. Also spitting of blood, hemorrhoids, and, especially in maidens, copious nose bleeding come from it, and endless other ills, which we think too many to relate." Even for his time, Marinello displays a penchant for exaggeration. The symptoms of menopause are diverse and the effects of declining hormones known to be extensive, but even without a medical degree I know for a fact that "spitting of blood" doesn't appear on any list.

Despite having been accomplished and necessary healers throughout history, especially regarding childbirth, women weren't often welcomed as medical experts, were usually barred from universities, and—if born in the wrong century—likely to be accused of witchcraft. Many an innocent with a good knowledge of herbal remedies spent time on a ducking stool, or worse.

In her pioneering book *Hot Flushes, Cold Science*, Louise Foxcroft explains that eighty percent of those put to death for witchcraft were female, and most were older women. For context, she reminds us that the Church said, "If a woman dare to cure *without having studied* she is a witch and must die," which put the lid nicely on women daring to proclaim themselves healers or midwives. Around 200,000 women in Western Europe were tortured or executed in the three hundred years up to 1750. Americans were more measured in their approach to women and magic; Foxcroft says that a mere sixty-one proceedings are known to have taken place in New England during the seventeenth century, for which, ironically, we must be grateful.

Of course, the most famous of these took place in Salem, Massachusetts, in 1692, where two-hundred-odd women were accused of witchcraft and some nineteen executed. Reading accounts of the "trials"—and I use the word with deliberate sarcasm—the women didn't really stand a chance, whether they bothered to protest innocence or not. One poor soul claimed that she had arrived on a broomstick and conversed with Satan. It's been pointed out that the majority of the women who died were past their childbearing years. Coincidence? I fear not. As Foxcroft said of Salem: "Postmenopausal women were particularly vulnerable as they no longer served the purpose of procreation. If widowed, they neither fulfilled the role of wife, nor were they protected by a husband from malicious accusations, and women who inherited property violated the common expectations that wealth should pass down the male line."

The idea that aging equaled a pact with the Devil was challenged by the English MP Reginald Scot. In *The Discovery of Witchcraft* (1584), he said that women were particularly at risk of being accused of the crime "upon the stopping of their monthly melancholic flux or issue of blood," as this made them "falsely suppose" that they could "hurt and enfeeble men's bodies." In today's language, that probably means that they had their own opinions. Scot, who should be retrospectively canonized, said that witchcraft didn't exist and that the women under suspicion were just old and poor.

To drag a lone positive from this seething quagmire of negativity, despite the concept of our blood being seen as disgusting, by the late eighteenth century, the idea of it being actively venomous was over. Now menopause was medicalized as a terrible illness to be feared and treated. Things were—I'm sure you'll agree—progressing.

Irrational and Sex Crazed: The Next Stage

Welcome to the nineteenth century. It's over 300 million years since we crawled from the seas, and over 300,000 years since homo sapiens got going, yet we're still no closer to understanding women's later biological life. Crucially, though, this was the age during which menopause was formally identified. Before you start calling hallelujah for wider understanding, this was also a time during which you were likely to be committed to a psychiatric institution for yelling at your husband. Such spurious reasons as "suppression of menses" or "time of life" were sufficient to trigger insanity and get you locked up (also "novel reading" and "politics," according to a list of causes of madness and subsequent admission to the West Virginia Hospital for the Insane between 1864 and 1889). Thankfully, women aren't still subject to such restraints—or I'd unquestionably be facing my golden years sporting a straitjacket in a padded cell.

It was a French doctor who coined the word "menopause." Charles Pierre Louis de Gardanne first came up with it in 1821 in his must-read book *De la ménopause, ou de l'âge critique des femmes* (Menopause: The Critical Age of Women). By 1824, it was in a French medical dictionary. The word itself comes from the Greek; *menos* actually means month and *pausis* means pause or cease. Put like that, of course it doesn't sound quite so dramatic. The French may have come up with that fairly bland term, but they also conceived *"l'enfer des femmes"*—"the hell of women"—and described menopausal women as *"des reines dethronées"*—"dethroned queens."

Although the Industrial Revolution was heralding "progress" by firing up its furnaces and mills, for women it was frequently the same old story. Many eminent physicians at the time postulated that women lived at the whim of their malfunctioning (for which they meant "penis-free") bodies, which entirely dictated mood, health, and sexual impulses. Woman was, as Carroll Smith-Rosenberg puts it in "Puberty to Menopause: The Cycle of Femininity in Nineteenth-Century America" (1973): "Not only a prisoner of her reproductive functions but quite explicitly of two tiny and hitherto ignored parts of that system—the ovaries. 'Ovulation fixes woman's place in the animal economy,' one doctor explained in 1880."

Menopause was finally discussed and included in medical textbooks, which you'd imagine a positive, and perimenopause—the crucial years before the final point—was now generally identified as the "climacteric." Medics were recommending pills and potions for the many symptoms (the monetizing of menopause had very much begun!), but the fact that medicine understood more about our physiology didn't necessarily do us any favors.

So, by the middle of the nineteenth century, doctors pretty much linked anything menstrual, ovary- or womb-themed with madness and hysteria, especially if you were drawing near to the end of your cycles. At no time were women more likely to become unstable, the men said grimly, than around this passage. As you lost your one useful purpose, you also lost your marbles and even your health. Therein an archetypal double whammy: as a woman, you were damned if you were having periods, but even more so if they were stopping. Obviously, I acknowledge mood swings, but these are not to be dismissed as end-of-life flailings.

"Insanity frequently occurs at the change of constitution," states the obstetrician and writer W. Tyler Smith in his 1849 article "The Climacteric Disease in Women; A Paroxysmal Affection Occurring at the Decline of the Catamenia" (as is so frequently the case, the clue is in the title). "I have no doubt that it is often owing to the climacteric paroxysms. Each paroxysm is a distinct shock to the brain, leaving behind it peevishness, irritability of temper and eccentricity." Another 1830s physician was adamant that menopause was a clear prelude to depression and death: "There is a predisposition to many diseases, and these are often of a melancholy character," he stated. Again, a potentially amusing misunderstanding of women's bodies that fails to raise a laugh, because we are still more likely to be prescribed antidepressants than have menopause properly diagnosed.

As well as being insane and ill, once menopause had us in its grip, we were ugly. Women, when they became incapable of conceiving, were viewed as becoming masculine and repulsive. In 1882, the English doctor Edward Tilt, who wrote the first English book dealing with "climacteric disorders" in 1857, said that you could spot a menopausal woman a mile off. "There may be a drowsy look, or the dull, stupid astonishment of one seeking to rouse herself to answer a question." There's also a tendency to sprout hair on the upper lip and chin (the latter a fair point, especially if you add testosterone to your MHT cocktail—of which more later!) and "An unusual habit of throwing off clothing and opening doors and windows even in winter."

Sadly, as we became more repulsive, physicians of the time again noted that we were also driven mad with desperate and strange desires. A small proportion of women find their libido off the scale in the last throes of fertility, but more generally this sounds like male optimism, though it was never considered a positive: "My experience teaches me that a marked increase of sexual impulse at the change of life is a morbid impulse," said the ever-cheerful Tilt.

And the way forward? Keep calm and carry on being domesticated for the good of our health, as Elaine Showalter points out in her book *The Female Malady* (although society continues to seem hell-bent on making that a challenge). It was felt that too much education for women, or trying to emulate the strength and ambition of men, could cause mental breakdown. Incidentally, the word "hysteria" comes from the Greek word for the uterus, *hystera*—naturally.

"Education, attempts at birth control or abortion, undue sexual indulgence, a too-fashionable lifestyle, failure to devote herself fully to the needs of husband and children—even the advocacy of suffrage—all might guarantee a disease-ridden menopause," says Smith-Rosenberg.

It's all our fault, ladies!

Cure or Kill

Because it was seen as a disease, menopause needed to be cured. Some of the therapies sound staggeringly foul—and far more dangerous and disconcerting than any hot flash or sleepless night. At no time were "cures" more thoroughly and horrifically investigated than in the late nineteenth century, when menopause was being explored as a medical condition. As with so many historical "medical" diagnoses I use the term "investigated" with heavy irony. I think the kindest word for the science explored is "experimental." W. Tyler Smith's patronizing tone is reflective of the era. "Heavy and prolonged sleep, particularly in the morning, exerts a marked influence in increasing the severity and frequency of the paroxysms," he says firmly. Far better you were up at dawn doing housework! Though beware . . . as a paroxysm is defined as "a sudden attack or outburst of a particular emotion or activity," which could, I suppose, be anything from a snapped "Screw you!" to kicking your physician in the shins.

As is so often the case with the "speculative fiction" about menopause, that was clearly written by a man with no idea that you can go to bed at nine p.m., sweat your way through most of the night, and wind up having had only three hours of actual rest. What menopausal woman wouldn't welcome a lie in, sleep deprivation being one of the myriad symptoms. But you can't help wondering if he simply had an eye on all the jobs that wouldn't get done with women spending their days just lying in bed feeling sorry for themselves or lusting after the opposite sex, despite their arid repulsiveness!

For those of you who, like me, can't get enough of his "insights," there's more: "All violent mental emotion should be carefully avoided," and "Stimulating diet and stimulating drinks should be used only with the utmost caution." He's just one small step away from advising that, post-fifty, we be put down. Tyler Smith also liked to get his hands dirty, and he particularly delights in describing with eye-watering and vampiric glee the benefits of bloodletting. Without going into too much detail, this involves applying three or four leeches to the cervical area. Further joyful solutions included ice in the vagina and cold-water injections into the rectum. From a twenty-first-century female point of view, the very thought of most of these "cures" would be enough for me to say quite firmly that I was just fine, free of all my feminine wiles (or should that be viles?), and promise to live out my remaining years very quietly, under the radar, so as not to disturb men any further with my offensive presence.

I'd argue that this is certainly one reason why we've got to the twenty-first century without clear illumination and focus on menopause. It's as good an explanation as any other for the silence surrounding this most compulsory of female evolutionary biological processes.

Incidentally, as is so often the case, any patient's experience of vaginal leeching remains unrecorded. I couldn't find any "tried and tested" reviews available from those subjected to Tyler Smith's treatments, but I suspect he would have fared pretty poorly on Instagram likes.

He wasn't the only medic pioneering seemingly sadistic, or just plain silly treatments. Edward Tilt also recommended some quite eye-watering solutions for our failing bodies. "Camphor . . . seems to correct the toxic influence which the reproductive system has on the brain of some women." Going one step (or staircase) further, he says that "In some cases of perverted cerebral innervation, the inhalation of chloroform, or of a mixture of chloroform and ether, may be usefully carried to the verge of unconsciousness." And who wouldn't like a vaginal or rectal suppository of opiates . . . Tilt also talks lightly of the application of leeches to the anus or ears. Or six to eight—count 'em—leeches on the perineum.

An especially sadistic-sounding expert named Dr. Isaac Baker Brown thought that the best way of sorting out female insanity (generally, not just in the case of pesky menopausal women) was by removing the clitoris. In five instances he operated on patients who wished to divorce their husbands, and lo and behold they returned to the marital fold. He was, you will be relieved to hear, removed from the Obstetrical Society of London in 1867, though far too late for his victims of female genital mutilation.

Less violently, surgeon Andrew Currier advocated simple problem-solving in the 1890s by whipping out the ovaries and thus causing menopause. In 1897 he also wrote the first book by an American physician to focus entirely on menopause.

There were plenty of such unnecessary-sounding operations performed, with an overwhelming air of "might as well give it a go" about the whole thing and a high degree of trial and error, but scant regard for patient safety or expert knowledge. Would such experimentation have been similarly indulged if it was killing off men, I wonder?

Although most of the surgical interventions of the late nineteenth century sound like the work of focused lunatics, there was some method in the apparent madness of these doctors. Occasionally, they'd pioneer a treatment that would result in a genuine breakthrough.

In the early 1890s, for example, a French scientist injected a menopausal patient with ovarian extract to cure her "madness," and three years later, in 1896, a German physician used desiccated ovaries as a "cure." These rudimentary experiments represented a step forward in the search for solutions. Today, MHT, or menopausal hormone therapy, is made from substances that mimic female hormones. As for information from women themselves, aside from occasional female perspectives such as Trota and Hildegard, there are few clues as to our thoughts on this singularly female experience. We see occasional shafts of light, suggesting that women were relieved to be free from periods and pregnancies, that older women might be useful within the family and at work, and that, once menopause was over, we might enjoy a peaceful old age. Never equal to men, naturally, but at least not entirely redundant. When your chances of dying in childbirth were so high, menopause must have come as a blessed relief for many of the sorority.

Moving on through the buckets of leeches and discarded organs, Judith A. Houck, in her brilliant 2008 book *Hot and Bothered: Women, Medicine and Menopause in Modern America,* says that both male and female (would you believe it!) doctors in the States were starting to rebrand menopause as a phase all women go through rather than black magic. "By the turn of the twentieth century, physicians increasingly offered their conclusions directly to menopausal women. Menopause started to be perceived as a phase, to be viewed scientifically."

What About the Women?

Excitingly, we were starting to see qualified female physicians. These women often disagreed—unsurprisingly—with the dramatic and ghoulish solutions and opinions of their male colleagues and took, on the whole, a far more pragmatic approach. Before 1847, women who wished to be doctors had to travel away from the States, but in 1849, Elizabeth Blackwell was the first woman to be awarded a medical degree. In 1864 the first Black woman to earn an MD—Dr. Rebecca Lee Crumpler—graduated from the New England Female Medical College in Boston. (In the UK the first female doctor was "allowed" to qualify in 1865—Elizabeth Garrett Anderson.) During the 1890s there were seventeen all-female medical schools, and by 1910 there were just over nine thousand female physicians—six percent of the total. After this promising start numbers fell and some of the women-only medical schools closed. But the point is that there were female doctors—frequently despised and harassed, obviously, but present, and with their very own views on their bodies.

Houck references the words of Dr. Sara Greenfield, writing in the *Woman's Medical Journal* in 1902, complaining that most textbooks only had a couple of paragraphs about menopause and that they "Dismiss it with the statement that it is a natural physiological phenomena which needs no special attention." To be honest, that sounds rather like today's medical training! The US was on the whole pretty sensible by the late nineteenth century— recommending healthy living, exercise, little alcohol, and (more bafflingly) avoiding tight-fitting clothes. Houck also points out that only twenty of the two-hundred-odd doctors writing about menopause during the forty years from 1897 onwards were female. Men generally wrote about it as degenerative and women were more likely to view it as transformative, so the lack of increase in female doctors during those years has done us all a tragic disservice.

Bottoms Up! What Were They "Thinking"?

In the early twentieth century, even the emergence of a promising new form of therapy, psychoanalysis, did women no favors. Sigmund Freud is perhaps most famous for his early-twentieth-century penis-envy theory, but he also said, "It's a well-known fact . . . that after women have lost their genital function their character often undergoes a peculiar alteration." Sadly, this personality change didn't provide a platform to object to men making unsubstantiated statements about our physiology. Freud further added, as though we hadn't endured enough, that women "become quarrelsome and obstinate, petty and stingy, show typical and anal erotic features which they did not show before." He must have been such a blast at dinner parties; I know I would have begged to be seated next to him! In fairness, it's not only men who have opined negatively about our journey into the next phase of womanhood. A student of Freud's, the psychiatrist Helene Deutsch, referred to menopause as—variously—"partial death," the "natural end as servant of the species," and a period of "psychological distress." She's actually right about the latter, but that's mainly down to the inexhaustible supply of gloomy mythology to which she seems to have enthusiastically contributed. Again, she would have made any book-club evening with the girls a lighthearted romp.

Our lack of ability to think coherently at this time of life meant that menopause could even be used in court. A paper published in 1999 covered this quite extraordinary subject. "Because of menopause, m'lud" was used from 1900 to the 1980s in the United States, and the "menopause defense" was actually taken seriously in some cases of divorce and serious injury. The first documented reference to menopause in a reported legal decision was in Texas in 1900, where a gas company (thankfully unsuccessfully) alleged that injuries sustained by a woman who fell into an uncovered trench were due to her menstrual problems rather than the fall.

Famous feminist Simone de Beauvoir was also pretty mournful about menopause (and aging generally), which she called "the dangerous age." Writing in *The Second Sex* (1949), when in her early forties, she pointed out that "While the male grows older continuously, the woman is brusquely stripped of her femininity ... Well before the definitive mutilation, woman is haunted by the fear of growing old."

Unhelpfully, she also focuses on the theme of us returning to girlishness, saying of the aging woman: "In a pathetic effort, she tries to stop time ... She ostentatiously brings up her memories of girlhood; instead of speaking, she chirps, she claps her hands, she bursts out laughing." This faux return to adolescence is referenced throughout nineteenth-century writing as well, and is just as patronizing and insulting as any "hysteric" label. Happily, once through the transition, she's a mite less pessimistic. "It has been far less somber," she pondered about aging in *All Said and Done* (1972), "than I had foreseen."

Staying Pretty in the Sixties

In the mid-twentieth century we struck gold, when hormone therapy became prevalent in the US. The time had come to enjoy the ride, ladies! Menopause was a deficiency disease, but no worries as long as you take the drugs. In the swinging sixties, MHT was all the rage, and in 1966 the American gynecologist Robert A. Wilson, who published a book called *Feminine Forever*, told us why. His unequivocal viewpoint: ladies needed to remain young and fun or they'd lose their husbands, and quite right, too. Neither young nor fun himself, Wilson charmlessly refers to the menopausal state as "living decay," with some quite staggering claims. Menopause is apparently a "curable disease" and also "completely preventable," and why wouldn't you want to stop it in its tracks, as "the unpalatable truth must be faced that all postmenopausal women are castrates." That's right. We're just men without testicles.

Interestingly, Wilson references his own experience, which included "the tragic decline of my gentle, almost angelic, mother . . . I was appalled at the transformation of that vital, wonderful woman who had been the dynamic focal point of our family into a pain-racked, petulant invalid." Wilson's book is still famous, and is referenced in histories of menopause, although he's not viewed as the helpful prophet I suspect he felt himself to be. Helpful to whom, one has to ask; certainly not the fifty percent of the population being misinformed and mistreated as a result of continuing levels of ignorance. It's useful if you want to be reminded how much worse attitudes toward women were last century, but otherwise, definitely not. There are days when I feel as though I exist in a state of living decay, but looking at the men around me is a welcome reminder that aging happens to us all, Mr. Wilson.

Most significantly, Wilson calls menopause a "tragedy." Poor us. "A woman's awareness of her femininity completely suffuses her character and . . . the tragedy of menopause often destroys her character as well as her health." On the bright side, he appears to be genuinely promoting education about the subject and trying to ease symptoms. However, describing menopause as a "mutilation of the whole body" is neither helpful nor illuminating. This sort of negative wording just adds Wilson to the long line of male observers of this specifically female phase who have no real idea what they are talking about. It seems relevant to add that Wilson's book was funded by a drug company, which may have added to his enthusiasm.

In the 1970s, in the second wave of feminism, there was a backlash, when us pushy women insisted that we, too, had a voice. We pointed out, with some vehemence, that menopause was just part of the natural process of aging, and it should stop being treated like an inevitable illness. "Even today the literature . . . defines menopause as a deficiency disease . . . It certainly echoes once more the male prejudice against menopausal and postmenopausal women," said a 1977 article. Women, on the other hand, argued that it could be rather marvelous. "Because menopause freed women from the risk of pregnancy, it was viewed as a sexually liberating event," said writer Frances McCrea in 1983. And yet, "The aging woman has a particularly vulnerable status in our society . . . To blame all the problems that aging women experience on menopause is a classic case of blaming the victim."

Has much really changed? The fact is that, until very recently, women have experienced menopause and men have had opinions about it. For hundreds of years it has been documented and treated by those who haven't had so much as a twinge of period pain, never mind experienced monthly bleeding, pregnancy, and childbirth. That's not to say that every observation made down the centuries has been incorrect, but many of them are, and the weight of all that toxic mythology is why we're in the undesirable place we find ourselves today. In direct contrast to the decline in our hormone levels, negative misinformation has continued to rise. If I have an agenda, it's to turn back the tide of misrepresentation that has overwhelmed my own sex with unnecessary fear and apprehension, as well as totally misleading the rest of the population about a natural, entirely survivable and potentially emancipating phase of our lives.

Today, over three thousand years on from Pharaoh Ramses II correctly pointing out that there was no point in trying to help a sixty-year-old woman conceive, and following four waves of feminism, one of the few absolutes for women, apart from death, is that we will experience menopause. Most recently perimenopause has entered common parlance as being perhaps even more significant than the moment itself. Yet both remain dirty words, avoided in conversation and still certainly not on the menu in civilized company. How are we ever to understand what's happening to our bodies when the outcome of centuries of propaganda is that we're often too ashamed to admit to ourselves that change is occurring? A friend's husband once described childbirth as "smarting a bit," a level of ignorance that sums up the problem with letting men's observations through the annals of time define women's experience.

In 1998, Phyllis Kernoff Mansfield, professor emeritus of women's studies at Penn State University, who has authored many studies about menopausal attitudes, asked the rhetorical question: "Why do women continue to feel they don't know anything about menopause? Because every woman's menopause is unique and no study has validated that uniqueness," thereby summing up the single biggest issue with how we treat menopause today.

In the next chapter, we'll talk about what the word actually means, but, in short, you are said to have gone through menopause on the twelve-month anniversary of your last period. Used to describe the potential decade of biological turbulence preceding that auspicious date, and the further fine-tuning that carries on afterward, it's misleading and even redundant. Using menopause as a catch-all term for every ailment a woman might experience from her mid-forties onwards is a classic example of the herd assumptions that continue to be applied to our sex. This natural biological progression, a waypoint that will affect each and every one of us in entirely different ways, is scooped up, mislabeled, underexamined, and misdiagnosed. Culturally and medically, it's regarded as an ending rather than a new beginning. It's high time we rallied together and refused to allow our functioning lives to be so unfairly foreshortened. Language speaks volumes, and the term "menopause" still carries a lot of deadweight. The end of our periods is the signal that we've been through a biological reboot, yet too often treatment only comes at the end of that passage. Most of us will need some support for the sake of ourselves, our families, and our careers. So why are we still so afraid to ask for it?

It's high time we renovated and elevated this life change. Despite the centuries of speculation and propaganda, we are not overheating or inherently cold, we are not hysterics or boiling vats of toxic poisons, we are not dried up or washed up, we are simply menopausal. Far from shutting down, having made that progression, we can open up to feeling freer, braver, and more liberated than ever before. Understanding what's happening and ensuring that our health, both mental and physical, becomes a priority is what will make it a story with a happy ending.

Small Men: The Clear and Present Dangers of Medical Sexism

The subject of bias in medicine is a necessary addendum to this chapter. This seems appropriate, as that's how women have always been perceived in medicine, as an "extra," an aside, or simply, as greater minds than mine have suggested, as "small men," rather than living entities that are glued together using different biology. This perception has hugely impaired and damaged treatment of women and it is a situation that's only beginning to be recognized and rectified.

Medicine is, and always has been, sexist, with the spare-rib theory informing medical attitudes since the dawn of time. There is a lack of female representation at every level of medicine, from patient to professor. It's only, shockingly, now, in the twenty-first century, that the health system is waking up to the physiological differences between the male and female body.

"There are decades of poor treatment and gaps that exist for women in medicine, and the situation is deplorable. We are not just small men," says Dr. Roxana Mehran, professor of medicine and director of Interventional Cardiovascular Research and Clinical Trials at Mount Sinai School of Medicine. Back in 2019 she co-founded the nonprofit organization Women as One, launched with the sole focus of promoting talented women in medicine.

She points out that there are a lot of female general medics—around fifty percent of the total who enter medical school and qualify—but many forms of bias make it very hard for us to progress.

"The road is long and treacherous, with steep hills and mountains and a lot of gravel in our shoes," she tells me. "Only eight percent end up in interventional cardiology and those actually practicing is down to four percent. Women leave; there is no quality of life, there is mistreatment and there are no leaders to follow."

There are only eight chiefs of medicine in the entire US who are women, which is hard to believe. "If you are a woman, working, sacrificing, and delaying building a family life while all the men keep climbing and getting the important leadership positions, why would you bother?"

Medical research is similarly unequal. In 2021, Professor Mehran authored a study into authorship of cardiology clinical trials revealing that only thirty percent of trials had women as the first author between 2011 and 2020, and many articles had no female authors at all.

The way in which women are treated in a medical environment is also of huge concern. Traditionally, drug research was performed on what was considered to be the average (of all humanity!): the 155-pound male. The bodies of women, with our hormonal fluctuations, were considered too unstable for testing, rather than greater concern being given to the absolute importance of ensuring that drugs (and dosage) were suitable for us. Generalizing and misinterpreting clinical data means that women's healthcare is compromised by a lack of understanding as to how drugs work in a more estrogen-rich (or depleted) environment. Women are, after all, up to seventy-five percent more likely to experience an adverse drug reaction.

A brilliant 2009 paper lists the physiological differences between the sexes when it comes to drug absorption. Women, it says, are not only governed by different hormones, but we also have slower gastrointestinal motility, lower body weight, higher fat stores, and more sensitivity to beta blockers, opioids, and SSRIs (selective serotonin reuptake inhibitors).

In 1993, the FDA issued a guideline for the study and evaluation of gender differences in clinical trials. This was to ensure that the safety and efficacy of drugs would be adequately investigated in the full range of patients who would use the therapy. Subsequently there was a whole flurry of papers investigating gender equality in clinical trials with, you will be unsurprised to learn, dismal conclusions.

Dr. Mehran says that the lack of senior female representation in hospitals is vastly impacting patient care. "We know that there is an important sex concordance in improving and enhancing the health outcomes of the patient. If a patient looks like the doctor and vice versa, then there's more chance of the patient following instructions and being more compliant."

There are so many ways in which the clinical environment is betraying women, with our "atypical" bodies. Women's pain is less understood and less likely to be taken seriously. There is a plethora of data backing this up—a 2021 analysis bluntly attributed it to gender stereotyping.

The very fact that Dr. Mehran saw a need to found her organization highlights the fact that the current status quo is outrageous, discriminatory, and needs to change. From our cradles to our graves, there exists a disastrous level of ignorance about female biological makeup. "Irrational," "angry," "hysterical," and "depressed" are just some of the words I've seen applied to women who were simply trying to navigate physiological turbulence during their body's metamorphosis. Medicine must acknowledge that women's bodies are very different from those of men, and that there's a need for women to have equity in the medical profession and medical care. It is imperative that we are taken seriously when we're going through hormonal free fall, specific to the female of the species, and one that affects us as much emotionally as it does physically.

CHAPTER TWO

A Road Map to Menopause

What is menopause? Well, for all the secrecy and overtones of doom, it's a pretty straightforward concept, and directly connected to its equally hot younger sister, puberty. First the hormones go up, and then, decades later, they come down again. Twelve months after your last period, you are said to have gone through menopause. That's all it is, just a day, or even a moment.

Except it's not. What we understand now is that in preparation for that defining end date to our fertility, there's up to a ten-year period of seismic hormonal activity we call perimenopause as our egg supply dwindles and hormones react accordingly. It's a turbulent phase for many women that experts now consider to be the time when we start to suffer the majority of symptoms caused by hormonal chaos. If ever there were a topic we need to "lean in" on, perimenopause is up there in my top five. Menopause needs to be on our radar and in discussion at least from the beginning of our forties.

The Starting Line: The Science

"We start our lives with all the eggs we are going to have," says menopause specialist Dr. Mary Jane Minkin, clinical professor in the Department of Obstetrics, Gynecology, and Reproductive Sciences at the Yale University School of Medicine, and creator and author of the excellent blog madameovary.org. "Simply put, in a standard menstrual cycle the estrogen made by the area surrounding the egg thickens the lining of the uterus. Mid-cycle we release the egg, ready to be fertilized. The ovaries also make progesterone, which prepares the lining of the uterus for the reception of the egg. If the egg isn't fertilized the progesterone starts falling. The trigger for our period is that fall of progesterone.

"In perimenopause, our supply of eggs is dwindling and therefore the manufacture of estrogen goes down." This is not, she warns, a tidy and linear process. "The way I explain it to my students, although these days they're too young to remember the banking crash, is by drawing a jagged line going downwards and explaining it as a terrible few days on the financial markets. That's what your estrogen production is like. Some days you're making none and others you're on double time and it goes crazy." When eggs aren't being released, progesterone production also declines. "That's why you get the crazy bleeding." Here, she's referring to the heavy periods in your late forties that many women endure and mistake as a sign of continuing fertility when in fact they're an indicator of impending menopause. Remember that although your fertility is decreasing it doesn't go to zero until you've gone a full year without a period. "I always like to emphasize that you can still get pregnant in perimenopause."

Although puberty has its mysteries, it's far more heavily investigated than menopause, and it's also a celebrated rite of passage, famed for the moodiness, pimples, parent-loathing, and door slamming that kicks off when the sex hormones get the business of fertility underway. Behaviorally, I'd say that it puts menopausal women in the clear, or maybe we've just learned better restraint by midlife! Menopause, of course, has no such celebration.

The Unmarked Path of Perimenopause

The confusing thing about menopause is that it's not a direct diagnosis, but a retrospective one. How can you possibly know twelve months in advance that it was the last time an egg plopped into the fallopian tube?—Instead it's almost certain it will go unnoticed and unmarked. It's all about the years before and after, and every experience is unique. One woman might have thirty hot flashes a day, another might not even notice the transition.

It's reported that eighty to ninety percent of women will have some symptoms before and after that menopausal moment. I'd say—based purely on my own observations over the last few years—it's more like a hundred percent. They may start a few months or years before and last an average of four years after menopause, but also might be as long as ten years before and twelve years or (far) more after your last period, which adds up to a good quarter of our expected lifespan. Incidentally, the oldest recorded menopause was said to have occurred at the age of 104, which seems both unlikely and a particularly low blow.

The accepted wisdom has been that perimenopause starts in your mid-forties. But perimenopause is the stealth pilot of the process. Most of us are unaware that the effects of seesawing hormones may have insidiously started in our early forties or even late thirties. And, fun fact, during perimenopause, estrogen may rise, or spike, by as much as thirty percent, before it finally plummets. It's no wonder these years are finally being recognized as a significant marker on our biological journey.

Around one in every hundred women experiences premature menopause or Primary Ovarian Insufficiency (POI), when the ovaries stop functioning or working properly before the age of forty; sometimes with no obvious cause or because of genetic disorders, autoimmune conditions, chemotherapy, radiotherapy, surgery, or another medical condition.

When periods stop between forty and forty-five, it's called early menopause and this affects five percent of women. The final curtain for menstruation has been said to occur on average at the age of fifty-one, though it is now starting to be recognized that Latinas and Black women are likely to be earlier. The latter finding is the result of far too many years of insufficient funding for female health research and cultural exclusion. In case you're interested, I was bang on fifty-one, like a high school over-achiever.

Initially, as in my case, changes may well be vague, and get gradually worse over time. It can be near impossible to know whether you are perimenopausal, grumpy, ill, overworked, in a bad relationship, or stressed and—knowing modern women—with a permanent and overriding sense of guilt that it's entirely, if inexplicably, your fault. That's why ignorance becomes our enemy. Without being aware of what we might be looking for, it can take quite some time to recognize what's actually taking place.

By the time we finally make an appointment with a doctor, whether it's a primary care provider, OB/GYN, or endocrinologist, we are often on our knees with exhaustion. Perhaps even more irritatingly, the moment you near fifty, every emotion you display is likely to be dismissed as being caused by menopause rather than perfectly justified dismay, displeasure, anger, or frustration.

Incidentally, a friend's more enlightened children, having heard us chatting about this book, are asking her, repeatedly, whether it "might be menopause" if she so much as snaps at them, or forgets where she put her car keys. "They are, on the whole, absolutely right," she says. "The problem is that I don't want to give them the impression that I am in any way governed by my hormones."

"Postmenopausal" has historically been the term for the years after the menopausal moment. But you are also, of course, menopausal for the rest of your life.

On Evolution

Menopause is one of the world's greatest mysteries. Humans were for a long time thought to be one of only two mammalian species who go through the transition, the other includes various types of whales: orcas, belugas, narwhal, and short-finned pilot whales—names that are only helpful if you take part in trivia games. In a breakthrough moment in 2021 it emerged that giraffes spend thirty percent of their lives in a post-reproductive state. Menopause? We'll take that.

There are all sorts of theories as to the purpose of being exempt from pregnancy in the second half of our lives. Much of the animal kingdom is destined to procreate from puberty to the grave, with death often arriving during childbirth, so we humans are pretty unusual in our extended post-fertility phase, where we have time to focus on pursuits not determined by our gender. Along with those whale communities, we are fit and well enough to live a full life for decades after our last period. Why should that be? Is it yet another flaw in women's makeup? After all, in 1969, Dr. David Reuben called menopause "a defect in the evolution of human beings" (sigh).

The least inspiring theory is that, historically, once we were unable to have babies, we would probably die anyway. As our baby-making potential came to an end, so did we, assuming we hadn't already expired from blood loss or infection during childbirth. But many historians remind us that the maximum human lifespan hasn't changed a great deal since classical times; the oft quoted "three score years and ten" is actually from the Bible. It's just that fewer of us used to achieve that age.

But other considerations skew life expectancy. From 1500 to 1800, early church records in the UK suggest that as many as thirty percent of children died before their fifteenth birthday, and more than a third of women are said to have died during their childbearing years in medieval times. Even in the mid-nineteenth century, infant mortality could be up to sixty times the current rates in both the US and Europe. You needed to survive being born and then avoid smallpox, diphtheria, tuberculosis, and whatever other ghastly illnesses took us down before vaccines were invented. If female, you also needed to pull through the horrors of antibiotic- and anesthetic-free childbirth on a frequent and unplanned basis, after which point you stood a fighting chance of getting to old age.

So there were plenty of women surviving multiple births and reaching their menopausal years, only to find themselves ridiculed in historical accounts as repulsive, brimful of poisoned blood that needed expelling, or, in extreme cases, being drowned in a pond or burned at the stake for perceived crimes against the patriarchy, like moodiness.

My favorite explanation of menopause is also the most likely. What's known as the "grandmother hypothesis" suggests that the reason we have menopause is because we are vital to society in later life.

Leading anthropologist Professor Kristen Hawkes's work on the subject has been groundbreaking. Forgive the fangirl tone, but speaking with her was like a teenager being granted an audience with Taylor Swift. She says that living well past menopause was a likely feature of *Homo erectus* (an ancient species of early human), meaning that it could have evolved over two million years ago.

In the early 1980s Professor Hawkes went to live with the Hadza Tribe in Tanzania, and her paper about hardworking Hadza grandmothers was published in 1989. At this time most anthropologists subscribed to the "hunting hypothesis," whereby men caught the food to support the tribe and keep everybody alive. And yet what Professor Hawkes witnessed in those months she describes as not only confirming the grandmother hypothesis but also explaining much of human evolution. And yes, it was all down to older women.

"East Africa is a similar ecological context to that in which our genus *Homo* evolved," she says. "We were trying to be invisible as we followed the Hadza going about their daily lives, and we noticed older ladies, whom I estimated to be in their sixties, foraging for tubers, and they were getting as many as the younger women."

Whilst observing the male hunters heading out every day, she says that their activity didn't quite comprise the child support we've been led to expect. "The archaeology is all these stone tools and bones of big animals, and so we thought that must be the story." In fact, the hunters were focused on getting big game, which had an average success rate of less than five percent per day. They were actually competing with each other for hunting reputations. "It wasn't about supporting the family, but wanting the other guys deferring to them. That's no way to feed the kids." A 2024 paper, based on 570 hours of direct observations of the hunters, and co-authored by Hawkes, further supported this: "Men's foraging was not consistent with the goal of paternal provisioning in these data." As with so much of women's work it may not be as self-aggrandizing as metaphorically spearing a lion, but putting tubers on the table is actually the real lifesaver.

As Professor Hawkes continues, it was actually the daily productivity of the women that fed the children. "You could see how well the kids were growing depended on the mother's work effort until she had a new baby. And then it was the grandmother's work, her foraging productivity, that mattered. Ancestral grandmothers aging slightly more slowly could subsidize more so postmenopausal longevity increased." So, our long post-fertile lifespan is thanks to the grandmothers passing on the longevity genes that co-evolved with shorter birth intervals. "Mom can move on and have the next baby way before the first one can feed itself because it's going to be subsidized."

Therefore, much human evolution and behavior can be attributed to the grandmother hypothesis—that we are as valuable post-fertility as we are during our baby-making years. "Babies are incredibly sociable because survival depends on somebody's engagement, whether that be mom or gran," says Professor Hawkes. "This is so different from the other great ape babies that start getting their own food before their first birthday as mom carries them along while still nursing." Humans have larger brains—greater longevity favors slower development, which results in a larger brain size—and it's also the reason why humans have long relationships whereby men "protect" women. This last occurred because longevity increased in both sexes, but old men are still fertile and that surplus of fertile men of all ages meant that men left more descendants by "proprietary mate guarding" (claiming "ownership" of women) as a mating strategy. "Our pairing habits are a big contrast with the other great apes. It's also why the world is run by old men," says Professor Hawkes. At last, a plausible explanation!

The evidence does seem pretty compelling. In 2012, Hawkes published a paper with a mathematical simulation of how this would have affected lifespan over the centuries. Many male anthropologists responded with something of a global-wide scientific sulk and emphatic protestations that "men contributed, too." Of course they did, but those efforts have been more than fairly documented! The grandmother hypothesis is, in a nutshell, what sets us apart from the apes, dogs, and cats. Postmenopausal women aren't going to take up time and resources having babies, so they can forage, farm, help raise families, or—these days—run global corporations.

Imagine this! Old women are useful! There's no chance that's making the headlines! I'm sure there are those who will cry, "Fie to such a feminist conspiracy theory!" But this is no speculative stab at a thesis, it's an anthropological conclusion based on compelling scientific evidence. Women are as valuable postmenopause as we were before, and it's clear that nature wants to keep us alive. Now we just need society to catch up with the idea. We need to start seeing our infertile later years represented less as a punishment and more as a gift to humanity.

The Information Maze

So how are we expected to find out about menopause? If you are reading this book, then you probably know that there is currently no standard path to illumination. My contemporaries may remember the slender books about sex and pregnancy handed to us by mothers in our early teens, probably rather furtively, back in the seventies and eighties.

I certainly wasn't aware of a similar step-by-step introduction for menopause, with easy-to-follow diagrams, but I'd be hugely grateful if my daughter was given one. For women now approaching or in the throes of menopause, knowledge is essential. Equally, for young girls, preparation for what's to come counts as a necessary part of the tool kit for life and can have a valuable impact on the choices they make about when to start a family.

Until recently, there's been no sense that women need any sort of literature or chat about the end of our fertile years, even though it's just as significant a process as the beginning. How has this happened, and especially in a world where we now talk openly about periods and our sex lives? You'd think that an automatic perimenopause meeting in your mid-thirties or early forties with a healthcare provider would be an obvious and positive step, like Pap smears and mammograms. It's certainly part of what we should be asking for when it comes to a new, enlightened approach to women's health.

There's a strong genetic component to menopause; you are very likely to follow your mother in terms of both timing and severity of symptoms. But such information may be extremely hard to extract. We polled a number of friends in their forties and fifties whose mothers—untruthfully, in most cases, we suspect—claim to have no memory of menopause at all, or point out that in "their day" you just got on with it and "there wasn't all this fuss."

In order to self-diagnose, you first need to have somehow absorbed the information that your anxiety, sleepless nights, forgetfulness and irritability, hot flashes, and aching joints might be signs of menopause and not just stress, depression, terminal illness, or incipient madness.

Next, you will probably visit Dr. Google (and discover you have symptoms synonymous with incurable cancer or a rare tropical disease), then phone a friend, or make a doctor's appointment, and at that point you enter a healthcare lottery as to whether you get clear medical advice, a prescription for antidepressants, or an opinion about MHT based entirely on your doctor or OB/GYN's personal bias rather than science.

What's more, there's the risk that you'll end up having far more tests than necessary, as menopause symptoms can be similar to other conditions.

"The typical woman will visit three to five doctors before she figures out her symptoms are perimenopause and not some kind of dementia or heart problem or sexual health problem—some of the many things women explore, not understanding it's all under one umbrella," says Dr. Mache Seibel, women's health and menopause treatment expert, author of *The Estrogen Fix* and editor of the online magazine *The Hot Years*.

The Muddle of Medical Training

It seems incomprehensible that end-of-menses education isn't a key part of medical training. But currently, the vast majority of American medical schools and residency programs aren't educating about menopause. A 2023 nationwide assessment revealed that only thirty-one percent of obstetrics and gynecology program directors who responded said there was a menopause curriculum in their program. The conclusion was that there's a real lack of menopause education, consistency, and standardized care.

"Lack of education in the US is probably one of the greatest areas of misunderstanding. Or myth-understanding," says Dr. Seibel. "The data simply isn't being distributed, and although the internet is a big source of information, a lot of it is wrong." He points out that not only is there a vast swathe of uneducated OB/GYNs who have no menopause training, but that once you get to primary care providers, there's an even smaller number with a specialty in menopause.

"As doctors, we're trained in pathology—to treat and try, ideally, to heal or cure," points out board-certified OB/GYN Dr. Shieva Ghofrany. "Suddenly, all of health care has been foisted upon us, without us having either the training or the time. We ideally need a more integrated system. In addition, we've patients every fifteen minutes, and you don't have time to delve in and talk to the patient."

A 2019 Mayo Clinic survey representing twenty US residency programs in family medicine, internal medicine, and OB/GYN showed that only 6.8 percent of residents felt they were being adequately prepared to manage menopausal patients effectively, including how to use MHT. Not particularly reassuring for the millions of women needing support.

In 2022, Stephanie S. Faubion, MD, MBA, director of Mayo Clinic Women's Health, wrote an excellent review entitled the "Menopause Management Vacuum" in which she pointed out that ingredients in the bubbling cauldron of chaos around the subject (our wording!) included a lack of teaching, an unprepared health system, and ongoing confusion around the safety of MHT.

And how does this on-paper bedlam translate to real-life experience? Well, in 2018 AARP (American Association of Retired Persons) surveyed over four hundred women to ask about their experiences with menopause. Forty-two percent said they'd never discussed it with a healthcare provider and only one in five had been referred to a menopause specialist. These are presumably the lucky ones who have healthcare. An appalling one in ten women in the US doesn't have health insurance, and they are more likely to be low-income women, women of color, and non-citizen women. More than one in five Hispanic, American Indian, and Alaska Native women are uninsured. We'll be continuing the subject of disparity later on, but it's a blatant fact that sociocultural and economic factors are associated with severity of symptoms. Meanwhile, according to a 2023 Mayo Clinic study, women aged forty-five to sixty are forking out an additional $24.8 billion annually on direct medical costs related to menopause.

The Menopause Society (an organization for medical professionals and women previously known as the North American Menopause Society) is doing sterling work; you can search for one of their certified practitioners on their website (as well as information about menopause; details are in our resources section). But at the time of writing this book there were fewer than 2,500 of these specialists available. Well over a million women are entering menopause every year, so the math doesn't add up, even bearing in mind that there will of course be other practitioners trained in menopause.

"I think the void created in the post WHI-era (a now discredited 2002 study that meant millions of women stopped using MHT) has created the perfect storm. There has been a lack of training and interest in menopause research in medicine, a lack of awareness within the community of women and practically no conversations among women," says Dr. Sharon Malone, OB/GYN, menopause expert, women's health advocate, chief medical advisor at @myalloy, and author of *Grown Woman Talk*. "So much of the field itself is dedicated to not getting pregnant, trying to get pregnant, delivering babies, and doing surgery that by the time women get to midlife and don't need these things, they've pretty much fallen off the radar. No one has the time to discuss the issues they will face in midlife and worse still, most doctors pretty much don't know how to treat them.

"Another problem is that women haven't been empowered to have these conversations with their doctors. There is the stigma and shame around menopause, perhaps because it is associated with getting older, as if losing our fertility somehow diminishes our value. Also, as women generally, and Black women specifically, we are taught that suffering is just part of the legacy of being women. And we tend to suffer through things when we shouldn't."

I need to point out that I am in no way slamming the medical profession. It's simply that a rethink in training on this period of women's lives, and one that is costing insurance companies a fortune because of misdiagnoses, not to mention the cost to women's long-term health and mental well-being, would seem imperative in the twenty-first century.

This brings me to another gaping void in the currently available information. One of the biggest medical scandals in history occurred in 2002, when the aforementioned WHI (Women's Health Initiative) study was halted on the basis that menopause hormone therapy (MHT) significantly increased the risk of breast cancer (I'm paraphrasing here, as we delve into it in chapter four). This led to MHT, the greatest and most effective tool we have in managing the majority of menopausal symptoms, being branded as dangerous for well over a decade. Millions of women stopped using it, and it's only now being correctly credited and used for rebalancing plummeting hormones.

Following that study (and various others around the time), debate raged over whether or not you were taking your life in your hands by succumbing to MHT, failing entirely to address the fact that by not taking it you were putting yourself in danger of other serious conditions including heart disease and osteoporosis, but the damage had been done. From 2002 onwards, if you took estrogen and then developed breast cancer, you might suffer the added burden of wondering whether it was your fault.

Meno-enomics

Quality of treatment for menopause depends to some extent on where you live and your cultural background.

For a start, if you are less wealthy, you have less access to care. As I said above, ten percent of women in the US don't have health insurance, and this group is also likely to be disadvantaged in other ways. "You might not have access to safe and effective treatments, but also to healthy food to ensure you're maintaining a healthy weight," says Professor Jewel Kling, dean of the Mayo Clinic Alix School of Medicine in Arizona. "And that's without getting into the concept of allostatic load (the cumulative burden of chronic stress and life events), where there is significant and mounting data that adverse childhood experience such as abuse impacts the menopause experience.

"Because of the barriers and misconceptions revolving around MHT prescribing, to address the need for symptomatic menopause treatment many clinics were set up post WHI with custom-compounding bioidentical MHT, and most of these treatments are not covered by insurance companies, meaning that the people who can afford those products (some can be up to $2,000 annually) are the ones who have access to them," she says. "Everyone deserves access to menopause resources and support; however, data shows that Latinas and Black women are less likely to be prescribed MHT."

Government intervention and community-based resources could help address these gaps, she says. "Clinicians need to be trained and to have an appropriate understanding of the benefits of MHT, and to recognize that it's still our first-line treatment for women who don't have contraindications and are early in menopause. Fundamentally, exposing the current state and then creating a space to talk about it can help lead to vital changes including equitable menopause care."

Professor Marcy Karin, Jack and Lovell Olender professor of law and director of the Legislation/Civil Rights Clinic at the University of the District of Columbia, agrees that inequalities are severe. "While Obamacare offers a healthcare option that's cheaper and better, there are still many whose only medical care is for emergencies. And that means that you are so far removed from the consults, advice, and potential support that are available to address peri or menopause."

Information is also less accessible in rural places. Here, telehealth might come to the rescue. Many of the excellent companies launched have a focus on (at last) women's health, including menopause. "There's a real role for telehealth," says Professor Karin. "Rural areas can be lacking access to doctors trained in the subject and who can see you when you have questions. In these cases, telehealth is the best and the easiest way to gain access to specialists."

The LGBTQIA+ Experience

There is little research or acknowledgment of the fact that not every menopausal experience involves cisgendered women in heteronormative relationships, and this is doing the LGBTQIA+ community a huge disservice.

"At the end of the day much of what we know about menopause is the cisgendered experience," says Professor Kling. "There are tools that we can take and individualize it to our transgender and nonbinary patients, to ensure that we're addressing their health concerns." But, she says, the most challenging part from the perspective of a clinician is the fact there's so little data to guide people. "We need to invest in research and do a better job of training clinicians to care for this population. In addition, for this population in particular, additional barriers exist including societal discrimination, prejudice, and policies that negatively impact LGBTQIA+ people where they may not even feel safe going to a doctor."

"In healthcare, any time you're dealing with a specifically gendered dimension of care, it tends to make LGBTQIA+ people more vulnerable," says Dr. Emily Allen Paine, assistant professor of clinical medical sociology (in Psychiatry and Sociomedical Sciences) at Columbia University. "When you pair that with standard healthcare experiences focused on women, aging, and healthcare, where concerns are dismissed as 'oh, it's probably menopause,' there's a confluence of different factors that basically create conditions in which assumptions are made about LGBTQIA+ people and that leads to discriminatory experiences."

Dr. Paine is primarily working with older adults who are trans and nonbinary people. "They have brought up the fact that there's no language for them. For example, a trans man who has a uterus and is experiencing the symptoms that we call menopause . . . there's no framework for him."

If people don't feel comfortable going to healthcare providers, it's putting them at risk of a late diagnosis for conditions they might be putting down to menopause.

Dr. Paine wrote a paper in 2018 about sexuality and midlife in which she discussed the fact that lesbian women aren't asked about their sex lives and therefore aren't getting the support they need for sexual problems.

Here, she says, menopause can go one way or the other. "It can be a less distressing time if they are in relationships where their partners are also going through menopause because it can be normalizing, and they can experience more understanding." But it doesn't always work out this way. "On the other hand, if both are having stressful and disruptive menopause experiences, it can be a double whammy."

Dr. Paine points out that it takes an average of seventeen years for research to be implemented in practice, and that healthcare professionals have little time and few resources. "There needs to be education, and what's called structural competency and cultural humility," she says. "You need to recognize that your experience and ideas and norms are not going to be the same as the person in front of you, and you don't have to be an expert in what they experience and value to provide affirming care. You just need to be committed to meeting them where they're at and not imposing your own cultural ideas."

For those struggling to be comfortable in the healthcare environment, she says that LGBTQIA+ telehealth companies, which provide virtual and affirming care, are to be commended. "I would affirm what many are already doing, which is to rely on their social networks in terms of finding providers and social support."

Racial Inequity

We wanted this book to be inclusive of everyone with an interest in perimenopause and the wider issues around menopause, but knew we would be remiss not to point out that there is racial inequity in lived experience, research, and support. Women of color tend to have more symptoms but less support.

Dr. Sharon Malone has spoken and campaigned widely on the topic. "A longitudinal study—the study of women across the nation (SWAN)—followed women for over twenty years, and they found a couple of things when it comes to race; that Black women tend to experience menopause about a year earlier, that their symptoms tend to be more severe, and their symptoms last longer." She reminds us that the average amount of time that women are symptomatic is usually about four to seven years. "For Black women it can be ten years or longer. Now that's a long time to suffer. And I think that part of it is cultural. Black women have the burden of suffering as an integral part of life."

A 2022 SWAN paper (Study of Women's Health Across the Nation started in 1994, with the aim of studying women's health and the menopausal transition)—"Disparities in Reproductive Aging and Midlife Health between Black and White Women"—reviewed the differences in menopause experiences and health outcomes. It's pretty shocking reading.

As the researchers point out, SWAN women were born between 1944 and 1954. The Black women in the study grew up in a society where institutional racism was embodied in law. Black women were more likely to have socioeconomic disadvantages during childhood, more adverse life events, were more likely to report events such as financial stress or experience of violence, and to have a greater disease burden when premenopausal or beginning the menopausal transition. Disparities such as access to healthcare continued long after the 1964 Civil Rights Act, and the paper suggests that structural racism is a major contributor to these.

So perhaps it is not surprising that Black women were fifty percent more likely to experience vasomotor symptoms (hot flashes), which were more frequent, bothersome, and lasted longer—10 years versus an average of 6.5 years in white women. Black women had a higher baseline allostatic load (eleven biomarkers of health) than White women—and were more likely to have diabetes, metabolic syndrome, and hypertension. Another SWAN paper about hot flashes shows that Hispanic women fall in-between, at 8.9 years, and Japanese and Chinese women have the shortest duration, at 4.8 and 5.4 years, respectively.

Further analyses point out that Latinas and non-Latina Black women experience more frequent hot flashes, sleep disturbances, and depression. Vaginal dryness was present in thirty to forty percent of SWAN participants at baseline, and was most prevalent in Hispanic women, among whom symptoms varied by country of origin. There's insufficient research into Asian American women, who are more likely to report pain, anxiety, and decreased libido, and there has also been very little research into the experiences of Native American women, though 2014 data showed that they were more likely to report hot flashes than other women.

When it comes to treatment of women of color there are further disparities. "There are a lot of assumptions made by healthcare providers—these may be unconscious bias in terms of whether or not a patient will accept therapy or whether they can afford treatment, which means that women of color are less likely to be treated for symptoms that adversely affect quality of life," says Dr. Taniqua Miller, board-certified OB/GYN and midlife/menopause health expert. A 2023 study looking at almost 66,000 women demonstrated that White women with psychiatric conditions and menopause symptoms were forty percent more likely to receive a prescription for hormone therapy than Black women. In a 2022 analysis of SWAN data, it was shown that Black and Hispanic women had the lowest uptake of MHT.

There is also weight bias. "According to CDC data eighty percent of Black women will be regarded as either overweight or obese based on BMI, which we know is flawed. So healthcare practitioners are also very biased in this sense," says Dr. Miller. She believes that, within this subconscious backdrop of weight and racial bias, Black patients in particular may be blamed for their symptoms and offered less effective strategies for management of symptoms, namely recommendations for dietary modifications or weight loss. "Effective treatment should be more holistic, offering lifestyle modifications along with evidence-based menopausal hormone therapy treatments that data has shown to make the biggest difference in symptoms."

What can be done? There needs to be a renaissance in how we look at menopause, says Dr. Miller. "You need to know your biases. That's one of the first things. If you look up weight bias and racial bias there's so much data there, and there are lots of programs to help people understand, and it's something we need to be constantly aware of. However, I find a lot of providers don't embrace [their own biases] because it doesn't feel good." In addition, she says that you need to make a pact with yourself to be constantly questioning decisions and treatment plans, rather than accepting them at face value.

We also need to create more inclusive environments, thinking about the way we write, the imagery, and the messaging on social media. "Are you writing through a singular lens, focusing on white, cisgendered women?" (I hope not.) "We need to create an environment where people feel comfortable and patients are able to see themselves."

Disability

For those who are neurodiverse or who have disabilities, there is often an added layer of complication. "Generally speaking, there may be different experiences for people who are disabled menstruators or people with disabilities in perimenopause and menopause," says Professor Karin. "There is a lack of research, including the impact of neurodivergency and perimenopause, and the impact of different types of disabilities and lived experiences."

"Learning disability is a very open area and there's very little talk about it," says Dr. Minkin. "There are specific needs; women with Down's syndrome often go through menopause earlier, but they might not be able to express themselves about what's going on." So far, she says that there hasn't been a lot of research. "But I think it's an area that will be coming up."

Governing Menopause

Ah yes, the government. Let me start by telling you about a commentary I found that discussed how the effects of *Roe vs Wade* are cascading into many areas of women's healthcare, including that of midlife women. It reminds us that three out of five caregivers in the US are women and on average they are almost fifty years old. "Access to reproductive health care and abortion services is likely to become increasingly difficult for caregiving midlife women," they point out. No government to date has yet said, "Let's focus on menopause." Given that fifty percent of their voters will experience it, this seems shortsighted to say the least.

Menopause clearly needs to be addressed at the very highest levels. And here, you'll be relieved to know, there is some movement. Women's health research generally has been glacial in pace until now. But Biden's 2021–2024 administration, whatever your political leanings, did begin to rectify the lack of investment (and lack of interest) in women's bodies. In 2023, President Joe Biden and Dr. Jill Biden launched the White House Initiative on Women's Health Research. On March 7, 2024, in the State of the Union address, President Biden called on Congress to invest $12 billion into women's health research. Then, just a few days later, on March 18, 2024, he signed the Executive Order on Advancing Women's Health Research and Innovation, which—short version—will expand and improve research into women's health.

In May that year—2024 was a big one for menopause—Halle Berry, who was memorably (and incorrectly!) misdiagnosed with herpes rather than vaginal dryness, joined a group of senators from both parties to push for legislation (the Advancing Menopause Care and Mid-Life Women's Health Act) that would put $275 million into menopause research and education. Berry shouted, "I'm in menopause, OK!" on top of Capitol Hill, to cheers from women everywhere.

In addition—so many gifts for us!—the Pregnant Workers Fairness Act was enacted in 2022. "It provides people with access to reasonable accommodations at work on the basis of pregnancy, childbirth, or related medical conditions," says Professor Karin. "However, in spring 2024, when the Equal Employment Opportunity Commission came out with their final regulations implementing the Act, menopause wasn't referenced as an example of a related medical condition, which would make reasonable accommodations for menopause much clearer, helping businesses know their obligations and workers know their rights to them, as opposed to requiring a case-by-case analysis." Perimenopause is, she says, mentioned in a footnote. (More about the workplace and menopause in chapter eight.)

But, she says, Title IX of the Education Amendments of 1972, which prohibits sex discrimination in federally funded education and educational activities, *did* mention perimenopause and menopause in their new regulations that came out the same month. "Discrimination based on menstruation, perimenopause, menopause, or their related conditions is sex discrimination . . ." This is the first clear federal regulatory statement to make this clear. "After years of silence, we had three important federal policy releases in one month!"

Just as excitingly, and also something that has garnered a great deal of media attention, was the presentation of the Menopause Research and Equity Act to Congress in 2023. This requires funds to be allocated to the National Institutes of Health (NIH) for the purpose of menopause research and funding. As a piece in Oprah Daily by Dr. Sharon Malone and Jennifer Weiss-Wolf points out, only around ten percent of the NIH's current budget goes to conditions primarily affecting women. "And an even tinier fraction was applied to menopause research," they wrote. "This legislation will elevate menopause to the federal research priority it deserves to be." Let's hope this is the case, and politicians do, at last, recognize the value in respecting half their voters!

Media and Menopause

Now, dismissive as I've been about the role of the internet peddling fake news and throwing up goodness knows what incorrect diagnostics, there's no question that many in the media have used their power for good when it comes to perimenopause and menopause.

One of the new powerhouses on the menopause front is Pilar Guzmán, editorial director of Oprah Daily. She says that it's only recently that menopause has been highlighted in the media. "Oprah tried to do this twenty-five years ago when she started to go through menopause, because she's ahead of everything—and she could not book anybody on the show to do it. No one in her age group was willing to go on stage and say, 'I'm going through this' or 'I struggled through this.'"

Guzmán says that greater openness today is due to a combination of social media changing the way in which we consume media—far more rapidly and with more storytelling, with news stories juxtaposed with influencers' tips on such platforms as Instagram—and the industry evolving to encompass mental health and more holistic solutions to problems. "What felt like a random or disparate collection of symptoms that didn't add up to anything became a sort of constellation all of a sudden."

Putting menopause on the menu became something of a mission. "In 2022, Oprah said we've got to do something about it. We both agreed this was the sort of topic that needed mainstreaming, that needed storytelling and that needed airtime. Our sweet spot as a brand, historically, is the intersection of storytelling and hard-nosed journalism. We think of these things as mutually exclusive, but they amplify each other. People can understand the science and the politics but when they hear the story it resonates and that turns into action. And so we taped our first big Life You Want class on menopause, with Gayle King, Maria Shriver, Drew Barrymore, Dr. Sharon Malone, and Dr. Heather Hirsch."

The class, you'll be unsurprised to hear, was a resounding success, and dedication to the subject has continued—an entire issue of the physical *Oprah* magazine was devoted to menopause. "We have a wonderful dialogue with our users and our readers, and they're very engaged. So we hear from them, and we hear their gratitude for naming the thing that they couldn't name themselves because we are all so stifled by virtue of being women."

So Here We Are

Thankfully, many women are making menopause big news. Celebrities such as Naomi Watts, Oprah, Michelle Obama, Gwyneth Paltrow, Halle Berry, Brooke Shields, Salma Hayek, Carla Hall, Stacy London, Tamsen Fadal, and Drew Barrymore have all spoken passionately about their stories, and the need for more conversation. Inspiring doctors such as Dr. Mary Jane Minkin, Dr. Sharon Malone, Dr. Mary Claire Haver, Dr. Stephanie S. Faubion, Dr. Kelly Casperson, Dr. Lauren Streicher, and many more are speaking out and educating women. Then there are campaigning and educating communities—our very own Menopause Mandate, Let's Talk Menopause, The MenoChannel, Red Hot Mamas, and, of course, The Menopause Society are all doing a sterling job.

But campaigners, opinion-makers, and influencers can only achieve so much, as Dr. Malone points out: "What I think we really need is a series of public health announcements. Some of this has got to come from the government. And I think we need to educate women so they know what's coming and when to expect it. We need to ensure that women have equitable access to support. But we also have to face the reality that there is a shortage of trained physicians who know how to treat menopause, and this shortage is particularly acute when it comes to communities of color and women in rural communities. So we have got to come up with a better way to democratize this process. I think the solution must involve innovations such as telehealth. I think that push really has to come from the National Institutes of Health not only in educating women but also in correcting the misinformation that they themselves are responsible for creating."

Ever since the Garden of Eden and its spare-rib theory, there's been the widespread assumption that women are physically lesser beings than men, and that we are assembled from their leftover parts. Unbelievably it's taken two thousand years on the Christian calendar to reach the understanding that women have our own, unique biology. For way too long we've been regarded as secondary components of human (men's) health, and female-specific conditions, aside from childbirth, in which the whole world has an interest, have been left relatively unexplored. This is why today we find ourselves in the frustrating position of trying to level up millennia of ignorance. There clearly needs to be more focus, training, and a roll-out best-practice policy for this issue, which has the potential to negatively impact the present and future health of all women from cradle to grave and particularly in midlife and post-fertility.

Perimenopause and the wider culture around menopause need to be given the same priority as our Pap smears and our mammograms, and we need a menopause update or health check so that we know to recognize symptoms such as sleepless nights or aching joints as a possible first sign of diminishing hormones.

Thankfully today a change in attitude is springing up slowly. Over the last few years, menopause has landed firmly on the agenda for discussion. There are an increasing number of excellent free sources of information and there is that escalating chorus of animated activists campaigning for education, laws, workplace acknowledgment, and more medical training. There is—in a nutshell—hope.

"The cliche that menopause is the worst thing that can happen to you is a bit exhausting."

OMISADE BURNEY-SCOTT, FIFTIES, FOUNDER OF BLACK GIRL'S GUIDE TO SURVIVING MENOPAUSE (BLACKGIRLSGUIDETOSURVIVING MENOPAUSE.COM), NORTH CAROLINA

A question I'm really tired of is "Why do Black women have a different experience?" Because it's like people are moving in the world with blinders and have no sense, or curiosity about the different ways that people are impacted by racism, or patriarchy or misogyny or homophobia.

When people ask this question they want you to say something magical and different. "Oh, this is the reason." Not your history. Not all your family's experiences. Not systemic oppression. Those are some reasons. And then I'm also wary of the question because I don't want it to turn into a backward entry into the idea that there's something inherently wrong with Black people and this is why we're challenged by our menopause experiences, and so I get really annoyed by that.

The cliché that menopause is the worst thing that can happen to you is a bit exhausting, even from people who are talking about it more openly and holding space for people to talk about it. There's still messaging that feels like, if you have a uterus and ovaries, let us help you navigate the worst thing that's ever going to happen. It's reinforcing a narrative that in my opinion is very much patriarchal. And I think that some of the internalized patriarchy that we have as women agrees with this; getting it is terrible. It's awful. And whenever somebody is sharing information, I try to use language that's honest, but not negative. Right? So it is dynamic, it can be challenging, and it is unique.

"Such heavy periods I slept on towels"

BETH, FORTY-SIX, RESTAURANT WORKER, OHIO

I've always had really bad periods because of my severe endometriosis, but the last three years they've been so erratic and heavy that I've been changing a super tampon every hour as well as using a pad and sleeping on towels. I said to my doctor I couldn't live like this for the next ten years.

So I had a full hysterectomy six months ago. My body feels great again, but we didn't have any discussion about going into instant menopause. My moods are all over the place and I'm hot flashing like crazy, especially at night, when I'm awake at least three times blazing hot, whilst my husband is freezing in the guest room. I work in a restaurant, where I'm supposed to be a ray of sunshine every day, but I repeatedly go from my normal freezing to blazing hot in seconds and stripping off layers. People are making fun of me, and I'm tired and crabby all the time.

"There's a lack of empathy for disability and neurodiversity."

JENNIFER CAIRNS, FIFTY-TWO, ENTREPRENEUR AND FOUNDER, NORTHERN IRELAND (PREVIOUSLY FLORIDA)

I have blood cancer and had treatment, which initially included twelve weeks of radiotherapy, that put me straight into menopause. It's hard to pinpoint symptoms, but I had massive fatigue and brain fog. I feel that in the States, medicine is a moneymaking exercise and the more doctors, referrals, and medication you get, the better. There's a lack of understanding around menopause here and in the UK, and especially when it comes to being disabled and neurodivergent. I'm doing a lot of work through my company, Lady Rebel Club®, where we're helping to initiate forward thinking toward women and other marginalized genders who are neurodivergent or disabled/PwD across the globe.

"My menopause was uneventful"

TOSH, EIGHTY-THREE, RETIRED ACCOUNT MANAGER, CALIFORNIA

It's been a long while since my menopause, but it was uneventful. My period stopped, which I was relieved about. I was born in California and we moved back to Japan after World War II, then lived in Hawaii, where my father was a Buddhist minister. After college I moved to California, where I worked and brought up my family. In the fifties, we never spoke about women's things. Even when I first got my period my mother just said, "Oh, I'm sorry you have to go through all that kind of thing."

"I felt no joy in life"

CLARE, FORTY-SIX, LAW PROFESSOR, MASSACHUSETTS

The first thing that I noticed was weight gain. Two years ago I went to the doctor for an annual physical and she commented that I'd gained weight. She was pretty low-key about it, but I laughed out loud, sharing that the only thing I'd changed in my habits since my last appointment was training for and running a marathon. A marathon! The next thing that got my attention was mood dysregulation. Like most of us, I've had episodic anxiety, but I suddenly found myself ruminating and even having intrusive thoughts, which was a new thing for me. I have a social work degree, and I thought, OK, I know these symptoms! Then I stopped being able to sleep—between two and four a.m. I'd lie awake, often keyed up about nothing. And finally, I started to experience depression that reminded me of being postpartum, where everything felt flat-lined. It wasn't even that I was affirmatively unhappy as much as that I couldn't feel joy. I had a hysterectomy after my third child was born, and although I kept my ovaries, I was told I'd probably have early menopause. When I thought about it, I realized that I also had hot flashes, nothing like the stereotype, but I was running hot. The final kick in the teeth was when I started to lose sensitivity in my nipples and clitoris, and I was experiencing vaginal dryness.

"Nobody could tell me I was perimenopausal"

TAMMY, FIFTY-ONE, COMMUNICATIONS, MICHIGAN

One thing I found strange was doctors. I had two doctors, both female, one in Florida and one in Michigan, telling me that I was too young to be going through perimenopause at forty-five. I asked to have my blood tested but they both said no, it was a waste of my money because I was too young. Then finally I went to a very reputable hospital and saw a male doctor who finally said that yes, I was perimenopausal, but that it was mild, and just to keep an eye on symptoms.

"I saw twenty-eight doctors in five years"

KATE, FORTY-FIVE, YOGA TEACHER, CALIFORNIA

I had a very early menopause at age forty-two with masses of symptoms. It's been very trying. Lots of other conditions came to light. It was very dark for a while, and I had better days than others. Age thirty-eight I was trying to have a second baby and my doctor was tracking my hormones for fertility, but said that perimenopause was indicated. I was still having cycles, but they became very short and then very long. Then I was diagnosed with endometriosis—pelvic pain has been a big piece of the story—and extraordinary brain fog, fatigue, and—most interesting—tachycardia (fast heart rate), especially with hot flashes. My autonomic nervous system was affected. I saw twenty-eight doctors in five years seeking answers. The biggest challenge has been weight gain because I just can't move enough.

"I bled out at a wedding"

SARAH, SIXTY, CRISIS COMMUNICATIONS CONSULTANT, TEXAS

In my late forties I had such horrendous periods that it was hardly worth getting dressed. The last straw came when I effectively bled out at a wedding. It was at night and an outdoor venue, but even so, when my male friend looked down and said, "What's going on?" I was horrified to realize that I was bleeding onto the ground. After that I had an ablation, which stopped the bleeding and was the best thing I've done.

At age fifty-five I was diagnosed with triple negative breast cancer and went through chemotherapy, radiotherapy, and a lumpectomy. Although triple negative is very aggressive, it's not fed by estrogen, and I was grateful that I didn't have to take Tamoxifen. I had just started on MHT in the form of estrogen and testosterone pellets and after treatment I continued with this, so I didn't experience the catastrophic menopause symptoms that others endure. I take part in a breast cancer fundraiser every year called Art Bra, where breast cancer survivors are models, wearing elaborate costumes that center around bras. The first time I was sent a checklist for the hotel it said "bring your fans," and I realized that the majority of women were on Tamoxifen and having hot flashes.

CHAPTER THREE

First Impact

One of the major challenges with menopause, from peri to post, is that nobody can tell you exactly when it starts or stops. Who in their fifties can recall with any accuracy when they had their last period? This makes it challenging for anyone wanting to mourn or celebrate the final passing of their fertility, and that big one-year anniversary of its demise. Those of you intent on performing a ritual for the end of your reproductive cycle will find it's not a date you can fix with any degree of accuracy, a bit like a politician elaborating on his involvement in a sex scandal.

Pinpointing the starting line for hormonal decline is equally difficult and frustrating, even though this is a time when the first indications of fluctuating estrogen might begin. The average age of perimenopause was said to be forty-five, but it's now recognized that symptoms may well start in the early forties or even late thirties; rather like the "average" age of menopause at fifty-one, it's an unpredictable timeline. A decrease in estrogen affects the entire body and brain, and there are tons of potential manifestations.

Every woman's experience is unique, and many of the signs aren't obviously associated with menopause, such as thinning hair and dry skin, even if you are informed and on red alert. I now know that there are at least thirty ways of recognizing entry into perimenopause; many websites cite thirty-four, which is now an oft-quoted number. Others say, rather vaguely, that there are "more than one hundred." As is already abundantly clear, factual evidence around this compulsory period of female realignment is sparse.

Of course, there are hot flashes, the ubiquitous sweaty, fanning-yourself-by-an-open-window menopausal cliché, and perhaps the most obvious sign of hormones going off-kilter. But the first subtle indications of declining hormones and the twilight phase of our monthly bleeding tend to go unrecognized by the majority of us.

So you might—or might not—suffer from insomnia, anxiety, tender breasts, brain fog, irritability, depression, joint pain, dry skin, itchy skin, acne, thinning hair, loss of libido, fatigue, burning mouth, gum problems, weight gain (especially increased fat around your middle), bloating, UTIs, headaches, vaginal dryness, incontinence, increased body odor, increased bruising, tinnitus, and palpitations. What a hoot, and that list is by no means exhaustive. I have friends who have referenced such random and obscure ailments as swollen eyes, boiling hot feet (but no other body part!), itchy scalps, and numbness in their extremities as being linked to their hormones.

There's some personal comfort afforded by that diverse and plentiful list. The surprising symptoms makes it less shameful that I entered my own menopausal moment unequipped with any of the knowledge I'm now enthusiastically sharing, and is probably why I've embarked on a "survivor's guide" with all the evangelical glee of a new convert.

My Experience

I am well aware that my experience is only the tip of the menopausal iceberg, or—more aptly—the summit of the simmering volcano that signals that our bodies are rebooting.

It's easy for me to sit here typing away, advising you to keep an eye on your biological clock long before it stops ticking. I have the smug satisfaction of having fumbled my way through the tunnel and emerged, blinking and triumphant, on the other side. The good news is, as we wake up to the toxic propaganda that's existed around this most natural of processes, we realize that it doesn't need to be a dark enclosed space at all.

It's likely that having spent my early forties making babies, I missed the worst ailments of the latter part of that decade, when many women's symptoms start to manifest.

Rather, in a positive pile-up of female reproductive activity, I managed to produce two children and traverse through menopause all in the same decade. It's a scenario which makes me one of an escalating number of women in the Western world. For compelling societal reasons including workplace inequality and financial penalization for our fertility, we are frequently embarking on motherhood perilously late. While the full stop of fertility remains steadfast at around fifty for most of us, the ability to get pregnant naturally diminishes from our mid-thirties. Inconvenient as it may be, it's a biological fact that it's harder to conceive as you get older.

To digress, but hopefully informatively, pregnancy, even in my early forties, was, unlike the next phase in my biological evolution, actually a pleasure. After an emotionally wearing and erotically dwindling twelve-month period trying to conceive, I sailed through the first gestation without incident and gave birth to a healthy little girl called Molly Mae. My son, Dan, born thirteen months later, was a surprise to us all, conceived just five months after his sister was born after a few too many margaritas on a Mexican vacation!

My first child seemed to provide the reproductive stimulation my body needed for round two. My second outing, apart from three months of an oily fish addiction, which on more than one occasion resulted in my husband returning home to find his baby girl crawling on the floor while her mother sat with sardine can in hand like a guilty addict, was otherwise also relatively uneventful. In fact, using my favorite bible, *What to Expect When You're Expecting*, there were few surprises that weren't detailed in that wonderful week-on-week companion to pregnancy.

Sadly, the menopause trek has no such predictable path. Perhaps it's because I had the two experiences of birth and menopause so close together that I am so acutely aware of the yawning chasm that exists between them in terms of knowing "what to expect."

Molly was only six years old when I started to experience the first hints of diminishing egg supply, but I had no idea that my experience was hormone related because I simply didn't have the information. If only the course of a woman's menopause were as predictable as that of carrying a baby, and there were easy-to-read and clearly diagrammed manuals. I'd love to see "irritability," "low libido," and "itchy eyes" depicted in a flow chart.

My initial menopausal symptoms weren't anything I might have been expecting even had I been better warned. They became palpable at the age of forty-nine, when I endured through two years of low-level anxiety and high-level insomnia before I finally had a diagnosis, and then, through MHT, supplements, and deep breathing . . . some respite.

Below are some of the main symptoms to be aware of, to which our menopause specialist, Dr. Mary Jane Minkin, offers brief solutions, some of which we will investigate further in later chapters.

Periods (of Change)

A good clue as to the state of your hormones are your periods, which are likely to become irregular; initially they may get closer together and then further apart, which is what happened to me. You may start to suffer PMS out of the blue or find existing PMS or PMDD is worse, and bleeding can be heavier, as the womb lining builds up more between periods. Or it may be lighter! Discharge may change in color and quantity.

Part of the previously mentioned SWAN study showed that ninety-one percent of women recorded between one and three occurrences, in a three-year span, of bleeding that lasted ten or more days, and seventy-eight percent recorded three or more days of heavy flow.

Dr. Minkin says: My friend Professor Nanette Santoro tells her patients that the uterus is like a lawn, with estrogen as the fertilizer and progesterone the lawn mower. This all goes awry in perimenopause. If you're in good health and a non-smoker, a low-dose birth control pill can regulate bleeding, and this may also help with hot flashes and night sweats. Or a progesterone IUD such as the Mirena can be placed in the uterus to give bleeding control as well as contraception, which is often still required in perimenopause. Maintaining a healthy weight is beneficial; generally the heavier you are, the worse your periods (fat makes estrogen). One can start MHT at this time but it is a bit trickier to monitor, as the woman's ovaries are still working, so you have to work in conjunction with them, often adjusting doses. As I always say, anyone can treat menopause—it's perimenopause that takes the real skill!

Regarding diagnosis, blood work during perimenopause can be of some assistance but is not definitive. Estrogen levels can vary from day to day. My patients often ask for blood work, which, by the way, is expensive, and I usually say: "If you are fifty-three, haven't slept a night in three months with hot flashes and your last period was three months ago, I don't need an estradiol level to tell you that you're heading into menopause." However, if

I have a thirty-five-year-old who has skipped a period or two and is feeling hot, isn't pregnant, and I've checked thyroid functions, then yes, I absolutely will check both her estradiol and her FSH.

Worrisome Times

Having never previously suffered from anxiety, I was completely thrown by debilitating and generally irrational feelings of trepidation. I had little to be genuinely stressed about, and yet there was no respite, and no filter.

I'd be as agitated about ordering groceries online as I was about getting home from another continent in time to relieve the babysitter. I just assumed that I needed to cope and get on with it, rather than wondering whether there might be a reason for my generally sensible self to regularly disintegrate into a seething mass of panic over what—rationally—I knew to be miniscule. For someone accustomed to seeing the bigger picture, and generally rising above ill humor or irritability in order to get things done, this was frustrating and upsetting.

There was certainly nothing special about my anxiety. It's said that over seventy percent of women may experience mood changes during menopause. That's very hard to pin down as a tangible "symptom," so you're unlikely to see your healthcare provider sitting back in her swivel chair and nodding sagely before scribbling a cure-all prescription.

I also had terrible irritability. Where my contemporaries had hot flashes I had rage flashes, with bouts of temper seemingly rising to the same unbearable heights as others' body heat. My teenage daughter insists that during this period I once threw a book at her! Luckily (if it actually happened) I missed, and, like childbirth, it's a moment I've forgotten, although it will doubtless feature, in a couple of decades' time, when she skewers me with her misery memoir of childhood.

What I do remember is two years of utter confusion and despair, wondering who the harpy in the house was and why, if my heart rate was any indication, even I was scared of her. Horror films about serial killers suffering terrifying divergent personalities (from *Psycho* to *Split*) briefly became an exercise in empathy as I experienced what it feels like when you become a total stranger to yourself. I think most women, however easy their periods have been, can empathize with the sensation of out-of-control hormones. Imagine feeling as you do the day before your period, but most of the time.

I found a study that I thought wryly amusing, suggesting that, for seventy percent of perimenopausal women, irritability is the main mood symptom, with researchers investigating what they called a "new, female-specific irritability rating scale." There were definitely days when I would have won top marks.

Dr. Minkin says: One of the major tricks is that menopause doesn't come at a convenient time and it doesn't announce itself. So how do we know if we're suffering life stress or menopause? Well, we don't. Anxiety and other mood changes tend to occur early on, and frequently women don't realize they're linked to perimenopause or menopause. I often say to patients in their late forties and early fifties, this is a time when your kids leave home and go off to school. Then, even worse, they come back! In addition, we're trying to break the glass ceiling at work, and we might also be looking after elderly parents (another laugh line for me: "even worse, mothers-in-law"), as well as dealing with marital relations.

For alleviating mood symptoms, estrogen therapy (MHT) is often very effective, and for those who can't or don't want to use this, you can try antidepressants—SSRIs (selective serotonin reuptake inhibitors) and SNRIs (serotonin and norepinephrine reuptake inhibitors) to help mood. Although there are some potential side effects such as a bit of weight gain and decrease in libido, these aren't usually a problem.

A holistic approach (which can be beneficial for many symptoms) includes managing stress, improving sleep, and a healthy diet. Cognitive behavioral therapy (CBT, see chapter five), mindfulness, and meditation may also help.

Hot or Not

When you have a hot flash, it's like nothing else, and you'll certainly recognize what it is! As previously mentioned I had the sum total of two, but I'll never forget the speed and strength of the heat that traversed from my feet to my head in a matter of seconds, making me feel like a latter-day Joan of Arc in her final crackling moments.

The hot flash is of course the classic and clichéd menopause symptom, and the one most likely to get you taken seriously. They actually have to do with the estrogen/brain connection. The part of the brain that controls temperature is called the hypothalamus. When estrogen levels go down, this becomes very sensitive to changes in body temperature and tries to cool you down via a hot flash—it's like internal central heating gone wrong. Anyone who has suffered such crescendos knows this is counterproductive, as you actually become scorchingly hot. More than eighty percent of us may get them, and for around twenty percent they can be disruptive to daily life.

Research now suggests that frequent and persistent hot flashes are associated with an increased risk of cardiovascular disease. Don't panic. Experts point out that this means there should be a focus on prevention in the form of lifestyle improvements and regular blood pressure and cholesterol checks.

Even my two flashes were memorable, with extreme heat hitting like a physical force. Of course, I suspected they might be connected to menopause, but then dismissed the idea because they weren't recurring, and like most women, I was very busy and forgot. To those of you suffering on a daily basis, I daresay the latter is evidence that mine really weren't that bad.

Night sweats are the nocturnal sisters of the hot flash, and they can ruin both sleep and quality of life. They occur for the same reason as hot flashes, but with the added indignity and inconvenience of occurring at a time when quality sleep is already hard to come by.

Dr. Minkin says: If someone patronizingly says to you, "It's all in your head," you can laugh, tap your forehead, and say, yes, actually it is. The most recent theory about hot flashes is that it's down to certain receptors in the hypothalamus, deep in the brain. These are called—collectively—KNDy (kisspeptin, neurokinin, dynorphin), and include what are known as neurokinin receptors. When there's a lack of estrogen these are activated, and this leads to a hot flash.

Hot flashes can last from a few seconds to a few minutes. Some folks say they last for hours, but this is very unusual. And they tend to get better over time, though ten percent of women have them for ten years or more. We don't know why twenty percent of women have none and twenty percent have very severe ones.

Solutions include MHT—you get estrogen therapy then you return to the old state of affairs. For those who can't or don't wish to take it, low-dose antidepressants—SSRIs and SNRIs—may be helpful. The one I like a lot is called duloxetine, and there's also paroxetine, citalopram, fluoxetine, venlafaxine, and gabapentin (which is actually an anticonvulsant). I run a clinic at Yale for cancer survivors, and I take care of a lot of breast cancer survivors, who can't or don't want to take MHT. We find SSRIs can be very effective.

There's new medication that blocks neurokinin activity. Veozah (fezolinetant) received FDA approval for safety and efficacy in the treatment of hot flashes in May 2023. This is also suitable for breast cancer survivors.

We know that lifestyle factors can affect hot flashes. Try to maintain as ideal a body weight as you can. Heavier women tend to have more— it's thought that extra insulation makes them worse (harder to dissipate the heat). Triggers can include caffeine, alcohol, and spicy food, and smokers go through menopause earlier and have more of a problem with hot flashes.

One of the oldest remedies is adding soy to the diet, which contains weak plant estrogens. This is thought to be safe, but check with your oncologist if you have or have had breast cancer, and make sure you eat whole soy foods; tofu and soybeans rather than extracts.

There is limited data on herbal products for hot flashes; there's some for black cohosh, and patients have found what's called Remifemin is good— this is derived from black cohosh. Try practical solutions such as fans in offices and bedrooms, wearing natural fibers, and CBT.

Be Still My Beating Heart

Palpitations may occur when estrogen drops, and they sometimes happen during a hot flash. Inconveniently mine tended to grasp me in the dead of night when I frequently found my heart rat-tatting like a machine gun. And of course we're less rational in the small hours, so anxiety can be exacerbated by the fear that your heart is about to explode from your chest.

I personally found that spreading my estrogen intake across the day, taking it morning and evening rather than all in one go, helped prevent the hormonal clashes that provoke palpitations, but let me step aside for the expert view.

Dr. Minkin says: Again, we think that palpitations are related to this hypothalamic activity, which triggers stress hormones that are released by the adrenal glands. Given the fact that there's often an increase in cardiac disease as women go through menopause, we usually encourage folk to have an evaluation, just to make sure we aren't dealing with anything significant cardiac-wise and then offer solutions—ideally estrogen from a hormone point of view.

Obviously, lifestyle is a huge factor in cardiac concerns. Look at coffee and alcohol consumption, don't smoke, maintain a healthy weight, and try relaxation techniques such as mindfulness and meditation.

Memory Matters

The inability to remember simple things, like the names of acquaintances, drove me to distraction. The brain fog of menopause can be pretty scary for those of us used to depending on our brain's ability to muster basic information. The sense of unraveling is only heightened when you lose the ability to bring certain words to the forefront of your mind, or find a blank space where there ought to be a memory. It may feel like you're in free fall but it's often down to simple chemistry. Estrogen is vital for both memory and concentration.

Again—and I have only just learned this, and found myself part of a large sorority in the course of writing this book—it's incredibly common. Some reports suggest that as many as sixty percent of women experience some form of memory issue around menopause. A 2013 study into the phenomenon, "Cognition in Perimenopause," showed that women in their first year postmenopause performed less well in verbal learning, verbal memory, and motor function than those in the earlier stages.

So yes, it is annoying to return to the house five times in order to remember everything I need, or popping out to the shops, staring blankly at the shelves for what I've come to purchase and returning with everything but the item I went there to buy. But I work on live radio, where lapsing into blank spaces when I'm counting on recall is terrifying.

Being a radio presenter, I rely entirely on quick responses, and short-term summoning of salient facts. These days, my preprogram notes are a forest-worth of illegible scribbles, as I jot down every thought, word, or phrase I might need to draw on later. We joke about becoming vague in our old age, but in reality, nobody finds it remotely funny. For previously swift and reliable recollection to diminish when you reach your mid- to late forties can be utterly alarming and discombobulating (I use the word mainly to prove that things do get better and vocabulary doesn't vanish forever!).

This means that far too many middle-aged women panic that they are showing early signs of dementia or that they're heading for a nervous breakdown. I know I worried about both. In reality, we just need to be aware that brain fog is frustrating, entirely normal, a passing phase as the brain adjusts to the low-estrogen environment, and that we might benefit from a top-up of estrogen, testosterone, more sleep, less stress, or just a simple recognition that our feelings are entirely normal, if unwelcome.

Dr. Minkin says: Brain fog comes back to the hypothalamus and is also probably related to lack of sleep. Estrogen can help, as can a healthy diet, good sleep, and exercise. Although estrogen is the ideal, in those who can't or don't wish to take it, I'm comfortable with prescribing a little Ritalin or something similar, though I prefer these patients to see a psychiatrist. People who had trauma early in life are more likely to have problems with brain fog. There's huge benefit in lifestyle approaches such as hydration, sleep (see chapter nine), and good diet (see chapter six).

Feeling Down

All feelings of depression around the time of menopause must be taken seriously. As with so many other related conditions it is hard to know where hormonal imbalance versus "normal" mental health problems interconnect.

As I've already mentioned, your GP may—often erroneously—prescribe antidepressants as a first port of call, and I was staggered at the number of women whose doctors refused to even contemplate a hormonal link between low mood and age.

We know that brain chemistry can affect mood. In 2014, researchers at the Centre for Addiction and Mental Health at Campbell Family Mental Health Research Institute in Toronto, Canada, identified elevated levels of a brain protein linked to depression, called monoamine oxidase A (MAO-A), in perimenopausal women. They suggested that this might help explain rates of first-time depression. MAO-A is an enzyme that breaks down serotonin, norepinephrine, and dopamine—the so-called happy chemicals. High levels of MAO-A have previously been linked to depressive disorders such as postnatal depression. In brain scans, this chemical was on average thirty-four percent higher in perimenopausal women than in younger women, and sixteen percent higher in perimenopausal women than in those in menopause.

More seriously, suicide rates are consistently highest in women forty-five to sixty-four years of age. The problem is very real.

Dr. Minkin says: Perimenopause and menopause precipitate depression in many women, particularly in women who have previously suffered from depression, including postpartum depression and premenstrual dysphoric disorder. And yes, there have been suicides. Perimenopause can really trigger things.

But the good news is that the depressive stuff tends to get better once you're through the transition. Women will often level out mood-wise once they are in full-blown menopause (with periods stopped for well over a year).

Estrogen therapy can be very helpful for depression, and for those who don't want to or can't, we use SSRIs and SNRIs—in lower doses. CBT, mindfulness, and yoga can be beneficial, and diet and exercise have been found to be helpful.

(Mariella says: Anecdotally, I was once prescribed St. John's wort in my twenties and it made me feel absolutely terrible, giving me palpitations and low mood at an age when I should have been in top form—so do watch out if you're trying to embrace "natural" supplements that have less robust evidence than FDA-approved medication.)

Breast Changes

Postmenopause, the breast tissue loses elasticity and may therefore become less, and I mean significantly less, pert than once before. Breast changes may also occur during periods and become more generally lumpy. As someone who has barely ever filled a B cup, my challenged mammaries may have been frustrating in the flush of youth, but at least there's not much to wave off now! Conversely, friends who are more bountifully endowed have complained that their breasts have become larger, inconvenient, and—they feel—distinctly unsexy. Proof, as though we needed it, that you can't please everybody all the time!

Dr. Minkin says: I don't know why breasts change and they often get bigger—you'd think that with estrogen going down, they'd shrink. I think some of this can be put down to perimenopausal weight gain. Some don't believe this exists, but I do—an average of five to eight pounds from the very beginning to the end of that magic year without a period. If you have any concerns about breast changes, see a healthcare provider.

Hidden Impact

Even if you don't have obvious symptoms, your body is still going to be affected by decreasing estrogen.

There can be silent damage caused by dwindling fertility hormones, such as loss of bone density and lack of protection from heart disease. A friend my age was fortunate enough not to experience any menopausal symptoms at all, and she led an irritatingly exemplary life, eating a plant-based diet and barely drinking. She was shocked to discover at a routine health screening at fifty-eight that she had osteoporosis and, despite her early misgivings, eventually embraced MHT, which has had a positive impact on her bone density.

It's well worth knowing that you can help yourself with these concerns, and we'll be looking at this in more detail in further chapters.

Dr. Minkin says: Even if a menopausal patient has no complaints, there are still health considerations that require attention. Both cardiovascular disease and bone loss are associated with the loss of estrogen. There are dangers from low estrogen that aren't necessarily going to be evident for some time yet.

Menopausal Migraines

I have never suffered from migraine but have enough friends who do—and who've found it increasing in severity, frequency, and duration around menopause, with thundering pain, vomiting, and days spent in bed in pitch darkness—to recognize the importance of the topic. The World Health Organization (WHO) categorizes migraine as a disability, and unfortunately it can often start or get much worse during menopause.

I asked Dr. Deena Kuruvilla, a board-certified neurologist and director of the Westport Headache Institute, about migraine related to menopause. "I'd say around ten percent of women going through perimenopause experience migraine, and it can begin from nowhere," she says. "Oftentimes, when a woman comes in and says she's developed migraine, she doesn't realize she's in perimenopause. Migraine comes with a variety of symptoms: dull pressure, pain, throbbing, sensitivity to light and sound, and nausea. One common misconception that almost every patient brings into the office is that if they aren't wearing sunglasses, sitting in the dark, or throwing up violently, it can't be migraine." She says in the vast majority of cases, as long as dangerous reasons are ruled out, that's what it is.

Dr. Kuruvilla explains that migraine is a headache disorder that occurs during overactivation of an area in the brain stem. This sets off a cascade of events where there's a lot of electric activity and changes to neurochemicals—culminating in migraine. Unfortunately, the estrogen fluctuations of perimenopause can be a culprit and for some women they can be completely debilitating.

Treatment-wise, specialists aim to preempt attacks rather than treat them once they occur, though emergency options would be offered if needed. "A lot depends on the frequency," says Dr. Kuruvilla. "Medications are a large part of the picture. If someone is having four or more attacks a month we might use beta blockers, blood pressure medication, antidepressant treatments like SSRIs or tricyclic antidepressants (e.g., amitriptyline), seizure medications such as topiramate, and Botox injections. There's also what's known as calcitonin gene-related peptide antibodies. These are drugs that block the specific peptide that's the main inflammatory factor in migraine.

"Some complementary and integrative medicines have science behind them, such as acupuncture, and we might add certain supplements such as magnesium, riboflavin, vitamin D, melatonin, and co-enzyme Q10 onto mainstream pharmaceutical medications or procedures.

"Lifestyle factors such as getting enough sleep, eating regular meals, and exercising all contribute to overall brain health and can significantly improve migraine," says Dr. Kuruvilla. "Have a high-protein diet and small healthy snacks in between breakfast, lunch, and dinner. Drink plenty of water, avoid alcohol, and try to do thirty minutes of aerobic exercise three to five times a week." She reminds us that stress management is a huge issue. "Self-care, mindfulness, and meditation can help manage stress, which can snowball and really contribute to migraine."

Dr. Kuruvilla says that estrogen therapy doesn't necessarily improve the situation. "While MHT may be recommended for many perimenopausal symptoms, it is not the first line of treatment for migraine related to menopause, and oral MHT has a small risk of blood clots. People with migraine have a higher prevalence of cardiac risk factors, especially if aura is involved."

If you experience migraine related to menopause, the good news is that there are many preventive and as-needed treatments to get you through the difficult time. Once you are on optimal treatment and have completed menopause, chances are that the migraine attacks improve.

Can We Blame Menopause?

Here is another problem, which flows seamlessly from the above concerns. I don't want to give the impression that all women over the age of forty are stumbling around, incoherent with exhaustion and rage but unable to articulate their feelings because of brain fog! That's not how it manifests. Work, relationships, and family will be prioritized and—usually—fulfilled perfectly adequately. The people punished tend to be ourselves as we take care of what we see as our essential responsibilities, forgetting that a well woman makes the world go around.

On this note, it may seem trivial, but I entirely blame my menopause for not having had the fiftieth birthday party to end all parties. With my anxiety levels and insomnia off the Richter scale, the thought of being responsible for a party to "celebrate" my five decades on the planet was way too onerous. Instead, as that auspicious birthday approached, I felt more like crawling under a shell than donning my glad rags and hitting the dance floor, as had been my intention in the preceding decade.

In the end, I was luckily rescued from my determination to stay in with my husband and young kids and hide from the world. I was overridden by my friend Amy, who refused to allow me that luxury and conjured a blissfully stress-free and age-appropriate surprise dinner party for a tiny group of friends at London's The Wolseley. When I look back on myself from my devil-may-care postmenopause prime, I barely recognize that shrinking violet. What a difference a few years on the right hormones can make! My fifty-fourth birthday, in contrast, was a raucous all-night party for two hundred, complete with live music, and my sixtieth an entire weekend of cavorting!

You may avoid symptoms altogether, but for those of us who don't, permanent exhaustion, irritability, and brain fog may feel as though they are impacting every single part of life, sapping the joy, destroying self-confidence, and removing the ability to perform as well as you want—whether it be at work or home—and affecting your closest relationships.

Now, in retrospect, I realize I'm one of many millions who suffered from unnecessary bewilderment and self-castigation, rather than what should have been swift recognition and diagnosis, both of which would have made life a whole lot better a whole lot faster. I'm so glad that thanks to small steps forward more women are entering this phase of hormonal turbulence better equipped with the knowledge that will ensure a smoother passage. Understanding what's happening to your body and eschewing shame and puzzled silence are instrumental in navigating your way into less turbulent seas. I am certainly no stoic, but because of my own ignorance and the lack of reliable information and support it took me two years to seek help and find solutions. My hope is that by reading this book you're on your way to a far speedier return to feeling like yourself again.

The Unique Experience

As I said earlier in this chapter, every woman's menopausal passage will be completely different. You are now hopefully better aware that symptoms are as varied as the weather and harder to pin down. For centuries the term "menopause" has been like a large black cloud hovering above our lives, obscuring attempts to better explore what for each woman will be an entirely subjective and navigable experience.

That's why this transitional phase in our biological lives needs individual and informed assistance to navigate, even if you're one of a small minority who notice nothing at all (in which case, I suspect you're unlikely to be reading this and best not to boast about it among less fortunate femmes!).

It seems obvious that attempting to deal with menopause as a universal condition to dismiss or "herd medicate" (I use the term ironically!) doesn't work. Yet still so many of us are left to flounder without proper care or assistance for perplexing symptoms. This entirely individual experience is seldom recognized as such in either the mythology or mainstream medical practice, and diagnosis relies heavily on our ability to intuitively recognize the changes occurring in our bodies and then demand the help and medication we might need. Listening to your body at this stage of life is imperative. Sadly—as many of us have found out—our own self-knowledge isn't always respected by the medical profession.

Do remember that your mother's experience is likely to be a good starting point for your own (so, if she's still around, I can't recommend strongly enough that you try to have the conversation). It's a maternal sharing session that's still all too rare thanks to the stigma, shame, and outdated societal expectation that a good woman should just gird her loins and "get on with it." Those myths have prevented better communication around our fertility journey but it's high time we liberate ourselves from them. The most valuable starting point for ascertaining what your perimenopausal journey may involve is your mother's experience, and especially when symptoms began (if she can remember). The added bonus is that it might also support her if you take the plunge when you're both young enough and open the door to engaging her on the topic.

"A future without children"

JODY DAY, FIFTIES, FOUNDER OF GATEWAY WOMEN AND AUTHOR OF *LIVING THE LIFE UNEXPECTED*, CORK, IRELAND

If, like me, you had wanted to have children, can you imagine the complexity of arriving at midlife without them? For involuntarily childless women, menopause is the end of any last smidgen of hope we might be harboring. People say it's not possible to "grieve something you've never had," but it most definitely is. It's called "disenfranchised grief" and it's a devastating loss—even more so as it's one that most people don't let you talk about, but instead close down your pain with trite responses.

The existential pain of childless grief at the same time as the final "full stop" of menopause can be so intense that I've referred to it as "a death you survive." It's a life-changing dark night of the soul that deserves much greater respect and sympathy than it currently receives in our grief-phobic and grief-illiterate culture.

I was forty-four and a half (those halves matter during your "still hopeful" years) when my second post-divorce relationship ended and I realized—finally—that I would never have children—that childlessness wasn't just going to be a chapter on my path to motherhood, but the whole story. The grief I felt was immense, although I didn't know it was grief at the time. Lots of us don't, and this, combined with the bias and judgments against women who haven't given birth is quite staggering. The "childfree" are those—approximately thirty percent—who have chosen not to be parents. But I'm one of the "childless," someone who wanted to be a parent and for whom it didn't happen. Fifteen percent of us are childless due to infertility, but many of us are childless by circumstance, such as not finding the right partner or being with a partner who doesn't want (more) children.

What I didn't realize as I started my grieving process was that I was already well into perimenopause. I am saddened by how ignorant I was for a well-informed and intelligent woman, as I would have made different decisions about my "unexplained infertility" in my marriage had I known. And as for "menopause"—I just thought it meant that your periods stopped around the age of fifty-one and involved hot flashes. I had never even heard the word "perimenopause" and was clueless about its complex and misunderstood symptoms.

If you are both unpartnered by a man and childless, once you hit menopause you are no longer part of the patriarchal project. You don't have the status of being a mother (or a potential mother), nor do you have the protection of a man's social position. When you consider that the only positive word in the English language for an older woman is "grandmother," you can begin to see this in action— all the popular in-use words for childless women from midlife onwards are insults, including "career woman," because whoever says "career man"?!

As a society, we don't need everyone to be having children, but we do need support for those who do, more acceptance for those who choose not to, and more empathy for those who are grieving that this is not the case for them. Adults without children contribute hugely and willingly to the civic society that other people's children rely upon—it's time to start seeing us as part of the human family, not as misfits. We matter, too—and so does our experience of menopause.

"Over a decade of hot flashes"

SUSAN, SIXTY-ONE, VOLUNTEER, FLORIDA

I'm very healthy, but I've been experiencing symptoms for almost eleven years, and it's horrible. At age fifty I had a hysterectomy and immediately went into menopause. I asked the doctor how long it would last and he said it could be a year, but it could be ten. It's been eleven now and it's still going. My mother took MHT and she had breast cancer, so I didn't want to use that. I took antidepressants for six months for my hot flashes, but they stopped working. Then I gave in and tried an estrogen patch, and that didn't really help. So I tried another antidepressant. You guessed it! That didn't work, and I still have them every hour to hour and a half. I just struggle through; they make me jump out of my skin every time and it really wears me down. I am frustrated and tired of having these flashes as a big part of my life. I started Veozah, the new, nonhormonal FDA approved drug, and it seems to help during the day, but not so much at night.

"We desperately need menopause education"

GABRIELLE, FORTY-FIVE, ATTORNEY, TEXAS

Imagine a condition where you may genuinely have thoughts of self-harm all of a sudden, but there's no advice available. Even in this information age and with such advancements in medicine, I have no clue if I am getting the best treatment. Perplexingly, hormones still seem largely a mystery to most doctors. I have PCOS (polycystic ovary syndrome), with fluctuating blood sugar and I get very hormonal around my period. I did not get diagnosed until I saw a specialist for fertility and that doctor actually performed an ultrasound on my ovaries. I now know PCOS causes early onset and longer onset of perimenopause, and I think I've been perimenopausal from around the age of thirty-seven.

"Wearing two bras for the breast pain"

CHRISTINA, FIFTY, HOMEMAKER, VERMONT

My symptoms started fifteen years ago when I was in my mid-thirties. I had hints that something was happening. I'd be fine and then have a week of night sweats and hives. Then about a year and a half ago the rubber really hit the road. I couldn't think, my body hurt, and I had terrible migraines that were getting worse. I had ferocious chest pains—as bad as when I was a teenager and my breasts were first growing. Everyone had to give me air hugs and I wore two sports bras every day.

My doctor said that I wasn't nuts and that lots of women my age go through this (!), and that the symptoms would disappear after menopause. I was offered MHT but I was nervous about breast cancer. Eventually things got so bad I had to cave in. I couldn't sleep any more, and the area between my legs was like sandpaper for a few days a month. Eventually I had some really long conversations with my doctor and decided to take it.

"The wicked witches were just going through menopause"

AMY, FIFTY-ONE, LEGAL SECRETARY, TEXAS

Those wicked witches in *The Wizard of Oz*? I reckon they were just going through menopause. Basically I've had all the symptoms except for hot flashes during the day. I was super depressed, I felt as though I had bugs crawling on my skin, I had migraines, palpitations, frozen shoulders, brain fog, low libido, night sweats . . . I used to be a good sleeper, but I was waking up all night.

And the weight gain! I've always been sporty and fit. I walk, I do Bikram yoga, and I've got ten menopause weight gain books in my apartment. I've tried so many diets but I'm seventy pounds overweight. I asked my doctor for advice and he said, "If you figure something out, let me know." Incidentally, he won't allow me estrogen because I still have my periods. I went to a hormone wellness clinic and burst into tears when the nurse listed potential symptoms. She was very Texan. "Ah honey, it's OK," she said, and put me on testosterone pellets. Within six months I felt better, but I could still sleep all day.

"I just stopped menstruating"

MARYLEE, SEVENTY-EIGHT, RETIRED DIRECTOR, OFF-CAMPUS COLLEGE AT CORNELL UNIVERSITY, MASSACHUSETTS

All my friends couldn't sleep, had night sweats, and mood changes, but I just stopped menstruating. I was about forty-nine and a widow. I'd been alone for seven years and had just started seeing someone, so I noticed when I got my period—it didn't come and then it did and was all spotty. I spoke to my OB/GYN and she said, well, that's menopause, and you might never see another drop.

"Not everything is menopause"

ASHLY BALDING, FORTY-FOUR, EXECUTIVE VICE PRESIDENT AND CHIEF SALES OFFICER, TEXAS

I think my story is a little bit different. In 2023, for six to eight months I'd been navigating extreme fatigue and migraines. I have two young daughters, I run a company, and I have to show up looking good. So I did every single thing you can imagine to keep me going. All my blood work indicated I was definitely in perimenopause, and then I got the hot sweats, which confirmed it.

Then a dear friend passed away in his sleep on October 26 and an angel spoke to me that night and told me to get to a cardiologist. I went a week later and they found a severe leak in my mitral valve. I wasn't getting close to seventy percent of my proper blood flow or oxygen. In December I had open heart surgery, spent twenty-three nights in the ICU and left with a pacemaker.

My experience has left me feeling as though we all need to talk about menopause a little bit more. But my message is that you shouldn't put everything in the menopause bucket. You can put a lot in there, but you need to get other things checked out as well, and younger women need to understand that things can happen to them, too.

CHAPTER FOUR

MHT

Part One: The Bad Rap

Back in 2002 the results of a major study stopped millions of women from taking menopausal hormone therapy (MHT), believing that it caused breast cancer. This meant that many suffered years of catastrophic menopause symptoms. Untold damage was done. In May 2024, a twenty-year follow-up revealed that these fears were largely exaggerated. This thankfully signaled a massive turning of the tides.

My appreciation of MHT is not to be underestimated. It restored my quality of life at the age of fifty-one, and has contributed to maintaining my state of health, hope, and (mostly) happiness ever since. There are—it's often stated—few certainties in life. But I'd add to the depressing clichés of death and taxes the absolute knowledge that, barring true disaster, such as global shortage, or a diagnosis that precludes it, I will cheerfully take MHT until I'm six feet under. My estrogen gel will have to be prised from my cold dead hands, which will still be clutching it the moment my soul departs from my body. That's how strongly I believe in its benefits. But whether or not to use MHT is hotly debated, and many of you will have heard the swirling inaccuracies that warned away an entire generation of women.

Without a doubt it is a decision that is, and absolutely should be, up to the individual and her doctor. But we can only make good decisions when we are armed with accurate information, and around MHT there remains a miasma of conflicting advice. As women we should have the right to make choices about our own bodies, but it's a right that many across the globe are still denied, and one that is curtailed in some parts of the US, where freedoms are sometimes seen being rolled back for one half of the population. It's an irony to cherish the right to bear arms, with the loss of life that all too often follows, but not our right to make decisions around our individual fertility.

So it's important to contextualize why we are still to this day unsure about the merits of the one advance that has a proven track record in mitigating symptoms of perimenopause and decreasing the risk of such serious conditions as osteoporosis and heart disease that can be prompted by our midlife hormonal freefall. Frustratingly, and despite overwhelming evidence to the contrary, there remains an ingrained fear that taking MHT might cause an early demise, in particular concerning the link to breast cancer, should you choose to supplement your declining levels of estrogen.

Memories are long, especially when it comes to health scares, and dirt definitely sticks. If you have qualms about the safety or efficacy of MHT, it is almost undoubtedly because of that 2002 report. At this time, a project known as the Women's Health Initiative (WHI) made global headlines when it claimed that estrogen-and-progestogen-combined MHT increased the likelihood of a multitude of health problems, including the risk of breast cancer. Until this point, it had been liberally prescribed, with around forty percent of menopausal women using it.

Google MHT and, to this day, thousands of websites still issue dire warnings, which are now years out of date. Thankfully, scientific opinion has shifted, and we are able to put those fears into context. For most of us, the benefits far outweigh the risks, but it has taken two decades to start undoing the harmful propaganda.

For clarity and better understanding let's take a quick trot through the development of this controversial medication.

The Toxic History of MHT

The development of MHT was conducted by men, whom it was suggested would benefit almost as much as the women for whom it was prescribed. Imagine the agony of living with a menopausal woman; all that flushing, forgetfulness, and dwindling libido. No man should have to suffer through that.

The first reported use of MHT to alleviate hot flashes was in 1897. The "modern theory of menstruation," as described by the Baltimore-born

gynecologist Emil Novak in 1921, said that the ovaries govern menstruation by secreting a hormone—a word coined in 1905 by Ernest Starling, a
professor of physiology at University College London, and which comes
from the Greek word *hormon*, meaning "to set in motion." A trio of men
isolated and purified estrogen from the urine of pregnant women around
1930; Edgar Allen and Edward Adelbert Doisy worked together in the
States, and German scientist Adolph Butenandt worked separately. Manly
handshakes, back slaps, and career prestige all around. Estrogen was, quite
rightly, perceived as a miracle substance.

Incidentally, the word "estrogen" also comes from the Greek. It is with
two raised eyebrows and eyes rolled all the way back in my head that I im-
part the knowledge that *oistros* means "mad desire" and *gennan* means "to
produce." Back in the day, it was no easy process procuring this precious
substance; in the 1930s, it took four metric tons of sows' ovaries to isolate
12 mg of oestradiol—a form of estrogen. Consider that a single pump of
the gel we rely on today is likely to deliver 0.75 mg of this precious ingredient. If, like me, you rely on two or three pumps daily, that's barely a week of
relief, and would call for the sacrificing of many sows. Then, in 1934, there
was further progress, when crystalline progesterone was isolated from the
ovaries of fifty thousand pigs.

I am simplifying the story enormously. There seems to have been quite
a race to work out what was going on, with a great number of rats and pigs
dying (and, presumably, a few female human casualties further down the
line) for the cause.

The commercial development of MHT began with the production of a
substance called Emmenin (sounds curiously like today's famous rapper,
though I doubt he'd be flattered by the reference) in the 1930s. This was an
estrogen product made from human-placenta extract and used for alleviating period pains.

Clearly, this wasn't an especially practical approach either; there is presumably a limit to how many human placentas you can lay your hands
on, so it must have been a brow-sweeping moment for women and the
drug companies when, around the same time, estrogen was found in the
urine of pregnant mares, and this was hailed as an easy and inexpensive
alternative.

In the early 1940s, the resulting drug, Premarin (from the words "pregnant mare urine"), was marketed commercially as an estrogen replacement in North America, along with early synthetic versions, though MHT wasn't available in the UK until 1965. Incidentally, Premarin is still widely prescribed, although there are newer forms available.

The (white, middle-class) reaction to such propaganda as Robert Wilson's *Feminine Forever* (the 1966 book extolling the virtues of MHT) meant that, by the mid-1970s, estrogen was the fifth most prescribed drug in the States. It was all rather Stepford Wives–ish; far less to do with our future health and far more to do with keeping us "fuckable."

There was a panic in the 1970s, when a clear link was discovered between MHT and endometrial cancer, but this was resolved by ensuring that all those with a womb also used a progestogen to keep the womb lining healthy.

The Scary Studies

That brings us to the latter part of the twentieth century and the beginning of the twenty-first century. There was strong feminist debate as to whether the use of MHT was ageist and sexist, but there were already noted benefits in terms of heart disease and bone health, and women taking it were said to enjoy a better quality of life. By the time things fell apart, around forty percent of menopausal women in the States were using MHT, and Premarin was the number one prescribed drug; sales of which were $1 billion in 1997.

"Hormone therapy has been around for over eighty years," says Dr. Sharon Malone. "So we have an enormous body of information and clinical data about the effects of hormones on women. Before 2002 I had been practicing for ten years and had been advocating that women take MHT, not just for symptomatic relief, but for the cardiovascular and bone benefits we had seen from years of observational studies."

Then the aforementioned 2002 catastrophe hit. Nothing gives a substance a bad name like a cancer association—though, on reflection, it's odd that many of us continue to smoke, drink, and eat unhealthy food in the face of very clear evidence that all have proven links. Unless you're a raw-food-munching vegan and have zero contact with twenty-first-century pollutants, chemicals, drugs, tobacco, saturated fats, ultra-processed food, or alcohol, MHT still isn't making it into any Top Ten "Steer Clear" list.

Doctors were aware of the possibility of an MHT/breast cancer link, but overall, studies were positive. The news that stopped the clock on millions of women overnight was the 2002 report by the Women's Health Initiative in America, when it was announced that researchers had halted the combined MHT part of the study early because women taking it were at greater risk of breast cancer, heart disease, stroke, and blood clots.

The headline on that initial press release read: "NHLBI Stops Trial of Estrogen Plus Progestin Due to Increased Breast Cancer Risk, Lack of Overall Benefit." It was a headline guaranteed to put fear in the heart of every midlife woman and that's exactly the reaction it got. Overnight, millions of women dumped their patches and pills. Doctors, no doubt fearful of lawsuits as much as their patients' health, stopped prescribing it. We women were, once again, on our own, left to cope with debilitating symptoms and long-term detrimental health impacts without so much as a cursory nod to developing an alternative. The problem was that the headline news simply wasn't accurate, and despite major concerns with how the study was conducted as well as how findings were interpreted and presented, the damage was done. There's irony in the fact that the Women's Health Initiative was launched in 1991 by Dr. Bernadine Healy, the first ever female director of the National Institutes of Health (NIH). And it's important to remember that the WHI has achieved a great deal of good. Even so, talk about the road to hell being paved with good intentions!

In 2017, one of the principal investigators in the WHI study, Robert D. Langer, MD, MPH, professor emeritus of family medicine and public health at the University of California, San Diego, wrote an article explaining that, when the initial results were assessed, most of the participating investigators, including several physician-epidemiologists like himself, were excluded. In fact, before he and his colleagues could intervene and make corrections, it had been finalized for publication.

He also said: "That headline, pandering to women's greatest fear—the fear of breast cancer—ensured that word of the study would spread like wildfire. And it ensured that the conversation would be driven much more by emotion and politics than by science."

We contacted Professor Langer to ask how he felt when he learned of the intention to publish the report. "I was furious," he says. "In fact, at the investigators' meeting when we were provided with the initial paper, I and several of my colleagues attempted to introduce revisions. That proved impossible as we were told the paper was already in print. Then, when we were shown the press release as a further fait accompli and told that it, too, would not be changed, I had a shouting match with the program director from the NIH, who was the first author of those materials.

"My primary point was that the intended headline was factually incorrect, extremely inflammatory, and irresponsible. I said that if the study was presented in that way, it would be impossible to have a rational discussion about MHT for years to come. I also pointed out that it was unethical to have submitted a paper in final draft to a journal, with named authors, including the majority of the investigators present at that meeting, who had not seen nor approved it."

Of the study itself, he says, "There was a problem with the ages of women enrolled." For example, the average age of the women taking part was sixty-three, which is a good ten years beyond menopause. "It is now clear that the response of major organs in women's bodies to estrogen changes as the levels decline. The fact is that maintaining levels beyond menopause with MHT is very different from reintroducing estrogen ten years later." In addition, many of the women were obese and half of them had smoked or were still smokers—both significant cancer risks.

"The most egregious flaw was that the harms touted for breast cancer and heart disease were so slight that they did not cross a pre-specified threshold for statistical significance," says Professor Langer. "In other words, it was scientifically wrong to say that there was harm."

(The MHT they were taking was a form of the pregnant-horse-urine estrogen [Premarin]. The vast majority of available research [both clinical trials and observational] reflects use of this form of estrogen, Professor Langer says. The progestogen used was medroxyprogesterone acetate, which is also still available.)

Dr. Mary Jane Minkin was practicing at the time. "Do I remember it? Absolutely. Did I know it was going to be a disaster? Yes. That morning I had fifty phone calls. The entire day was crazy." You cannot, she says, underestimate the fear of breast cancer.

"I was interviewed for the *New York Times* about it in 2023 and told the journalist: 'I remember where I was when John Kennedy was shot. And I remember where I was when the WHI findings came out.'"

Imagine, if you will, how different the landscape would have been had Professor Langer and his colleagues been allowed to make changes. He was absolutely correct in his predictions. Use of MHT plummeted by around eighty percent in the States in the subsequent years, but the damage went way beyond this. "It wasn't just research into MHT that stopped," says Dr. Minkin. "Everything stopped. Not only were women terrified of using estrogen, but we stopped teaching menopause management in residency programs. If you trained in the US post-2002, chances are you've got no education in menopause." This, of course, is why women in their forties and fifties are going to doctors with no experience in the subject. Terrifying, isn't it? "Even in my institution, where I make plenty of noise, I had to fight to get a lecture thrown in here and there."

To give you some context, a 2013 study of OB/GYN residency programs showed that only twenty percent (of those who responded) reported a formal menopause curriculum. That's a fifth of medics studying something that fifty percent of the population will experience. The math doesn't add up. A poll in 2023, despite all the myth-busting that has taken place, had this number creeping painfully to just over thirty percent.

These aren't simply numbers. They represent every woman who has crept up to me and asked for advice about her crippling menopausal symptoms. They're every woman who has endured hot flashes and bone deterioration, memory loss, vaginal dryness, hair loss, and unfamiliar aches and pains, all because a misguided report told her what would happen if she sought hormonal support.

Subsequent studies—including ones done by the WHI—have shown the clear benefits of MHT, but we (and the medical profession) have clung to the MHT = Breast Cancer equation. Funnily enough, headlines correcting the initial findings and taking a more balanced view never appeared, or at best were only to be found buried at the back of health sections of newspapers and websites. Corrections are not sexy or sensational. Headlines reading "MHT is actually OK" didn't have the same attention-grabbing potential, so millions of women remained (and remain) convinced that MHT imperils their well-being.

I was over the moon when a twenty-year follow-up was published in May 2024 proving that these fears had been mostly exaggerated; the *Washington Post* covered it, but basically, unless you were in the menopause world, it went virtually unmentioned.

"I believe that women who have gone through menopause since the WHI [report in 2002] have been harmed, and in many cases left to suffer with poorer health because of the unwarranted degree of fear stoked by the WHI," says Professor Langer.

"To be clear, MHT is not for every woman, and it—like any medical treatment—is not without adverse effects. The problem is that those adverse effects have been blown far out of proportion to the clinical and scientific reality. Moreover, it has led to the rise of many substitutes that have their own adverse effects, none of which are as good physiologically as estrogen to address issues that women in this phase of life might wish to treat.

"Not all women have indications for MHT, but for those who do and who initiate within ten years of menopause, benefits are both short term (relieving hot flashes and painful intercourse) and long term (bone health, coronary heart disease risk reduction).

"It is time to get past the misinformation and hysteria generated by the highly irregular circumstances of the WHI [report] and stop denying potential benefits to women who may be helped," he states. "MHT is appropriate for symptomatic women within ten years of menopause who have no major contraindication. Good evidence from over fifty years of observational studies and clinical trials suggests that the benefits outweigh the risks for most women when started early. I remain passionately committed to restoring rational discourse on this hugely important topic."

"During the twenty-two years since the Women's Health Initiative came out we lost a lot of ground," says Dr. Sharon Malone. "Not only in what women suffered through in those twenty-two years, but we've lost two decades in research. And now we've gone around the world and back again.

We advocated for MHT use not just for symptoms, but also for prevention of osteoporosis and heart disease. All of that went down the drain after the WHI. We're back now and we're just reexamining that data to admit that— You know what, maybe the WHI didn't say what we thought it said."

The Comeback

Aside from the millions of women who were frightened off taking something with the power to protect them from unnecessary suffering, the further negative legacy of that WHI report was that it stifled additional research. "Products went out of production and companies were worried about developing further options because of the stigma," says consultant gynecologist Janice Rymer, former vice president of the Royal College of Obstetricians and Gynaecologists. Menopause is a massive industry, with thousands of consumers entering every year, but nobody is going to make drugs that women are too scared to take and with publicized "dangers" that might make them liable. Easier to ditch the research and development and leave half the population struggling with the debilitating effects of managing menopause and its damaging effects.

Slamming shut the MHT door also opened all manner of opportunities for desperate women to turn to unscientifically proven solutions, searching for costly and unproven options elsewhere.

In the UK, the official guidelines were finally rewritten in 2015 to incorporate MHT as a first-line therapy for menopausal symptoms. In the thick of my own perimenopause at the time, I wrote about what a positive impact MHT had had on me, genuinely believing that the debate was over. The reaction I got from that piece, with total strangers stopping me on the street to ask whether they should take MHT, made me optimistic that change was occurring. But in subsequent years, while making my BBC documentary and researching this book, it became clear that many women are still absolutely fearful of side effects and don't understand the nature of the minimal risks, compounded by the fact there's confusion and ignorance even in the medical community.

MHT use remains shockingly low. At the Menopause Society annual meeting in September 2024, an analysis of insurance claims data revealed that although 4.6 percent of women over forty used it in 2007, this had declined to just 1.8 percent in 2023 (3.7 of women aged fifty to fifty-nine). Don't forget, not all insurers cover MHT. This didn't include custom-compounded hormones (see page 99), but it was pointed out that these wouldn't add more than a percentage point or two. And that 2024 follow-up is at least likely to mean a very welcome swell in physicians prescribing MHT, and women—at last—starting to feel safe about using it again.

The Brave Shame in Taking It

Rather like natural childbirth, over the course of history women have been given the impression that suffering is their lot, and those who eschewed support, like refusing an epidural, were somehow "better" or more virtuous for accepting the pain. There is no other human experience presumed to reward those who refuse the very thing that will improve their symptoms. Among the emails I have received since my campaigning around meno-pause began, there are still an overwhelming number of women who say things like "I'm wary of taking MHT," or "I know it's not fashionable to take MHT, but it helps me," as though it's a shameful reliance. Supplementing your diminishing hormones isn't on a par with choosing to wear knee-length when miniskirts are in. Of course it should be a personal choice, but one based on factual evidence and available information. Absolutely no one should be telling us what to do unless they have a convincing medical reason to put us off. Menopause is a topic of discussion that's all too heavy on rumor and low on tangible facts.

Acknowledging the Risk

Experts globally concur that for most women the benefits of MHT out-weigh the risks if taken within ten years of menopause or before the age of sixty—within what's known as the "window of opportunity." It can be started at any time, but it's better to begin sooner for bone and heart benefits.

"There is no increased risk of breast cancer with estrogen alone," says Dr. Minkin (this is only an option if you don't have a womb). With estrogen and progestin, the official number attributable is eight cases per ten thousand women per year over the age of fifty and after more than five years' use. It's now thought that the small breast cancer risk is associated with the older, artificial progestogens. With micronized progesterone now available, early studies are suggesting that there's no increase in breast cancer cases and even a possible decrease within the first five years of use. There is no increased risk of breast cancer mortality associated with MHT. Typically, none of the latter has been the subject of joyous rejoicing media headlines!

You are more likely to develop breast cancer from excess alcohol than MHT; my past enjoyment of wine may yet catch up with me. Drinking more than two units a day (around a glass of wine) is associated with five extra cases in every thousand women aged between fifty and fifty-nine. The greatest breast cancer risk is having obesity, which is associated with an extra two or three cases in every hundred women over the age of fifty.

None of this means that it's your fault if you develop cancer. They are risk factors, not predictions. Lifestyle changes can help lower the risks, such as cutting down on alcohol and being a healthy weight. There's less point dabbing on the estrogen gel, and more risk to your health generally, if you smoke and drink. Exercise can actively reduce cancer risk—there are seven fewer cases of breast cancer per thousand for women who work out for at least two and a half hours a week.

Dr. Minkin points out that there is a risk of blood clots from oral (tablet form) MHT. "It's a small event, perhaps one or two in a thousand. As we get older these risks increase, so many doctors switch people over to transdermal gels or patches."

In a 2017 Mayo Clinic survey of twenty US residency programs, thirty-four percent of residents said they wouldn't recommend MHT if a woman had severe symptoms even if there were no contraindications. Most of the women to whom we spoke hadn't even had a conversation about it or were warned off by cautious doctors.

Let's also remember that there are women dying from *lack* of MHT.

In the arid desert when it comes to investment and interest in women's health, we have to be grateful for glimmers of interest and information. A 2013 study from Yale University estimated that, in a ten-year stretch from 2002 onwards, over ninety thousand hysterectomized women may have died prematurely from not using it.

Far be it for me to preach (OK, I preach), but everyone needs to evaluate the facts and make their own personal decisions. I'm still staggered by how the negative spin on MHT has prompted so many women to feel it's a support they should resist rather than investigate further. And I'm infuriated that, if we do make the choice to boost our declining hormones, it doesn't necessarily follow that we're given what we need.

As with so many aspects of menopause, your opinion of what you need is valid. Most importantly, MHT ought to be automatically offered around perimenopause, along with all other possible solutions and lifestyle advice. Armed with facts, we are able to make judgments about risks versus results. The medical profession needs to have more confidence in diagnosing and understanding what's happening to our bodies. Until society catches up, we need to clue ourselves up on what's available and trust our instincts in terms of what we need.

Cancer and MHT

So, can you use MHT after cancer? In the majority of cases, the answer is yes. "Although oncology saves lives, it doesn't consider post-cancer menopause," says Dr. Minkin. "Women feel uncomfortable asking their oncologists about quality of life because of course they're thrilled to be alive." Fifteen years ago, she started a very successful program for cancer survivors, helping them to improve post-treatment life.

"Menopause as a result of cancer treatment (either chemotherapy or surgery) can come with the same symptoms as standard menopause, but often these start abruptly because of the abrupt removal of estrogen," she explains. "There can be hot flashes and night sweats, emotional and cognitive changes, sleep disruption, vaginal dryness and bladder discomfort, dry skin and hair loss as well as joint achiness." This might all seem like adding insult to injury—having gone through cancer treatment, you have to also deal with the challenging aftermath. "The most important thing to remember is that we have lots of options."

There are also, she explains, further day-to-day concerns. "Many will have had surgery and are dealing with changed body image. We have a psychologist as part of our team, meeting patients to see whether they need help with self-image or relationship issues.

"Most women who have had cancer and been rendered postmenopausal are candidates for MHT, as long as the cancer wasn't hormone sensitive, and especially if they are younger and therefore at significant risk for heart disease and osteoporosis in the future," says Dr. Minkin. "Cancers increase coagular ability, so we tend to recommend transdermal MHT (in the form of a gel or patch), which doesn't have a risk of blood clots.

"Most gynecological cancer patients can be treated with both systemic and vaginal estrogen—radiation to the pelvis can cause scarring and stenosis of the vagina, as well as vaginal moisturizers and dilators."

Then there's breast cancer. There are around 250,000 cases every year in the US. It's highly unusual for breast cancer survivors to be recommended MHT as there's always fear of recurrence and there isn't sufficient clinical data on the subject (for more information on this, I'd recommend reading Avrum Bluming's brilliant book *Estrogen Matters*).

The good news is that there are masses of other options for symptoms such as hot flashes. SSRIs and SRNIs are appropriate and effective, gabapentin is good for hot flashes, and will also benefit those with neuropathy from chemo. "Oxybutynin is appropriate for an overactive bladder and works for hot flashes, too, and fezolinetant is a new drug which is good for hot flashes," says Dr. Minkin.

My co-author, Alice, had breast cancer in 2023 (a very small triple-negative tumor) that was treated with chemotherapy and radiotherapy, and her oncologist didn't recommend that she continue with her MHT. She is now reluctantly experiencing what she calls a "second menopause," and is raging at the injustice of late-onset hot flashes.

"We need women to have access no matter where or who they are"

TAMSEN FADAL, FIFTIES, MENOPAUSE ADVOCATE, EMMY-AWARD-WINNING
JOURNALIST, AND AUTHOR OF *HOW TO MENOPAUSE*, NEW YORK

The twenty-year follow-up of the WHI that occurred in May 2024 is changing the way we perceive MHT, and kickstarting a revolution in it being correctly prescribed by doctors to all the women who are able and wish to take it. I lost my mother to breast cancer, and all the doctors were like "I don't know, maybe it's OK to take MHT but it's up to you." When somebody says that to you as a patient, they're very scary words, and I was afraid of it.

In 2019, I suffered a hot flash, palpitations, and brain fog in the studio to such an extent that I had to leave the set. I went to my regular OB/GYN who wrote in my patient portal, "In menopause, any questions?" and then I saw five different doctors.

Then I did my research—as a journalist that's what I do. I came across doctors who really explained it to me, and one in particular, Dr. Sharon Malone, whom I interviewed for my 2024 documentary, *The M Factor*. Then I was like, what am I doing? I've still got all these symptoms, I'm talking to all these women about this and I'm not doing it for me. So I went back to my doctor and I've been on the patch and progesterone ever since and it's made a huge difference.

But when I say to women that I'm taking MHT, I hear, "I'm not taking that. It causes breast cancer," and that's a singular fear for women. You ask them if they're afraid about heart disease, and they say, "That's something I'll deal with one day." Ask if they're afraid of dementia and they say, "I'm taking vitamins." Often we don't even think about osteoporosis. But breast cancer is such a fear, and I understand that because I lived with that cloud over my head for a very long time.

There still aren't many doctors who feel comfortable talking about hormones and MHT. So when we are educating women, we're saying go talk to your doctor, but then they show up at the doctor who isn't sure what to do, shrugs, tells them that MHT isn't safe, and puts them on antidepressants. Now you have double confusion! We need women to have access no matter where or who they are.

"I'll take it forever"

SANDRA HOWARD, BARONESS OF HYTHE, EIGHTIES, LONDON

I have always felt far more comfortable having MHT than not. I'm a doctor's daughter twice over and I don't believe in scare stories; I'm rather fatalistic. I had an early menopause, aged about forty-four or so, which was a disappointment, as I longed to have another child. My lovely GP eventually had a look at me and said, "You really aren't going to like this, but you will get such pleasure from your grand-children." I went straight onto MHT and am still on it. I never had any conscious symptoms, but the MHT gave me a feeling of slight confidence that I wouldn't dry up in all directions! One or two doctors have tried to suggest I do without, which I did try for six months. It might have been psychosomatic, but I feel far happier having it. I'm generally more bright-eyed, and my hair and nails are in better condition. Right now, I'm fortunate, as they seem very happy for me to carry on with a low dose, and I fully intend to stay on it.

"MHT has never been mentioned"

LINDA, FORTY-NINE, TEACHER, CALIFORNIA

I saw my OB/GYN when I was forty-one and asked whether I might be in perimenopause, but she said I was too young, and that was it. I felt very dismissed. I imagine from my weight gain and overheating that I'm now in the thick of things. I especially notice when I'm cooking dinner and I'm visibly too hot. I'll ask one of my sons to pass me the fan. I also worry about my poor memory and whether it's down to perimenopause or early Alzheimer's. It's a time of confusion and isolation. All I've been told is that I have high cholesterol. MHT has never been a conversation, but I grew up in the UK and Mum was on it, as are many of my friends.

"Breast cancer treatment threw me into menopause"

CASEY, FORTY, BOOKKEEPER, CALIFORNIA

I wish I'd known more about menopause before it was forced on me by six rounds of chemo for breast cancer. After the second round of chemo my cycles stopped and by the fifth round I had a deluge of symptoms: hot flashes, brain fog, interrupted sleep. I already felt as though a rug had been pulled out from under me, and all I was told is that many women experience menopause after chemo.

My team has been really sweet, but I've been told that they'll manage things as they come—the actual wording was that they'd "play whack-a-mole" with the symptoms. I can't take MHT because my cancer was estrogen positive. To be honest, I'm done with drugs; I've adjusted my diet and am the queen of cruciferous vegetables. I don't know why we're not generally given more information about how diet and lifestyle can help with symptoms. It would make a huge difference to millions of us.

"My HT isn't covered by insurance"

MARCELLA FARMAN-DIETZ, FIFTY-TWO,
EXECUTIVE DIRECTOR OF EVENTS, NEW YORK

I'm going to start MHT but my insurance—which is the top tier and costs $900 a month—doesn't cover anything but the pills and not the patches and the gel, which is what I want. And as for testosterone—forget it—insurance won't cover that. My doctor is trying to get me the combination patch, otherwise I'll be forced to take the pills. It's outrageous that the only options are synthetic. I'm not sure the problem is so much obtaining MHT if you push for it and advocate for yourself—doctors in the States are only too happy to hand out medication—but it's getting it covered by insurance, which is incredibly unfair and means it's only available to those who can afford it.

"I thought I was having a heart attack"

TESS STIMSON, FIFTY-THREE, WRITER AND JOURNALIST, VERMONT

At age forty-one I went from feeling absolutely fine to having panic attacks in the middle of the night that were so horrendous I thought I was dying from a heart attack. I'd wake up drenched in sweat with my heart racing at a million miles a minute. I've been in plane crashes, shot at, and had a really bad divorce, but nothing compared to this. After a few days I went to see my doctor who said I had anxiety and gave me Xanax and antianxiety meds that I took for about six months. But I didn't like the side effects so I came off and the attacks started again.

It had occurred to me that it might be hormones, so I went to see a nurse practitioner who said to suck it up and get on with it. She was really horrible to me. Eventually when I was forty-three I went to see a menopause specialist, who was really nice, and said that panic attacks aren't spoken about much but are quite common. She gave me estrogen gel and within three weeks I felt like myself again.

"I don't want to stop using it"

MARIE, SIXTY, HOUSEWIFE, DELAWARE

I didn't struggle in my forties, but I was on low-dose sertraline for depression, so I wonder whether that might have helped me through perimenopause. But then aged fifty-three things really started and I had hot flashes every night so that my sheets were wet and I'd have to change my nightshirt. My legs got very thin, in an unhealthy-looking way. We've all heard the stories about MHT and I assumed that I shouldn't take it, so I struggled on for three years and then went to the doctor at age fifty-six. It took a bit of time to find the right one and now I'm on the gel, with total relief from the hot flashes. Every now and again I stop to see whether I still need it, and they come flooding back. My doctor wants me to stop, but I'm very reluctant.

"I just wanted to understand the hormones"

CLARE, FORTY-SIX, LAW PROFESSOR, MASSACHUSETTS

When I called up OB/GYN practices and asked to speak with a doctor who specialized in menopause they were like "All the doctors can handle it." I live in Boston, a city full of world-renowned healthcare centers, and I went and had a completely underwhelming experience in terms of the doctor's curiosity and evaluation. I asked about progesterone and testosterone and she was dismissive. She talked about starting me on a low dose of estrogen but didn't explain why or what that does. She started to lecture me oddly on how much of the "management" would be "lifestyle changes." She started talking about an app to use, to I don't know what exactly—initiate sex or masturbate? I hadn't mentioned anything about my sex life being a problem. It isn't. She said I shouldn't drink anything before bed so that having to pee doesn't wake me. But I hadn't mentioned my bladder waking me. It doesn't. I'd talked about random sleeplessness and weird anxiety at night. She said to sleep in a very very cold bedroom—"your husband should be freezing."

By this point I'd had enough. I was so irritated. I'm a lawyer and a social worker. I'm well educated. I'd done my homework on managing what I could on my own. I said, "I'm going to stop you. You're making so many assumptions. Assuming I'm married. Assuming I'm married to a man. I mean I am, but you haven't asked me one question about myself. I'm here because you're an MD. I can google all of this. I want to know what the science is and what the hormones *mean*."

Part Two: MHT Love Song

There is no cure for menopause, because it is not a "disease," and I'm not sure "estrogen deficiency" is quite the right term either, with its negative connotations. But when you're going through a catastrophic loss of hormones, it seems sensible enough to try to top them up, which is why the term "HRT" seemed the most appropriate. Now we have the still-further abbreviated HT (hormone therapy) or MHT (menopausal hormone therapy), which make even more sense. Thankfully, discussing all these issues counts as progress, so let's not get too hung up on the details! Whatever solutions you choose will simply mitigate to a greater or lesser degree the impact perimenopause and menopause has on you.

"MHT replaces the two key hormones made by the ovaries: estrogen, which affects every organ in the body, and progesterone, to protect the womb lining," says Dr. Minkin. "Ovaries also make testosterone, but this is more of a gradual decline."

There are women who swear by MHT, women who swear they'll never take it, women who can't take it, millions who simply don't know what to do, and a further cohort who've never heard of it! The inclusion of testosterone may come as a surprise: yes, we have that, too. A neighbor stopped me in my apartment building the other day, a sophisticated woman in her mid-forties, asking if we could have a chat about her possibly perimenopausal symptoms. When I asked if she was on MHT she replied "What's that?," thus articulating clearly how far we still have to go in sharing knowledge and delivering support. To add to the confusion, healthcare professionals are similarly divided, though I have to say that every single menopause expert to whom we have spoken (bearing in mind they have specific and specialized training in women's health) was absolutely committed to its positive effects. Every single one. The global consensus is that for most women the benefits outweigh the risks.

However, not one expert has recommended eye of newt and toe of frog boiled up in a cauldron at midnight and ingested by the light of a harvest moon, nor any of the extraordinary, unproven, and staggeringly overpriced "remedies" available on the internet. MHT—and I acknowledge there are risks—has at least got countless *scientific* studies proving its efficacy.

In 2014, following two years of enduring my own undiagnosed and exhausting symptoms, I was finally prescribed the first version of the nonalcoholic cocktail on which I now thrive: transdermal (absorbed through the skin) estrogen, initially in the form of patches, which I didn't like, as they failed to break through the barrier of my body lotion, so I changed to gel, which did the trick; micronized progesterone, in the form of a tablet; and testosterone cream. Perhaps not overnight, but over a matter of weeks, the agonies of insomnia and the misery of being trapped in perpetual illogical anxiety faded to the back corridors of my memory. I was, to all intents and purposes, my old self, and I welcomed her. She had been absent for quite a while.

I suppose I may seem a bit gung-ho when it comes to medication, as a misspent youth means that there are few drugs I haven't tried or cocktails I've turned down. Obviously, I'm not advocating a party lifestyle. One of the pleasurable aspects of speaking to a more mature (I assume) audience is a sense of diminished personal responsibility. We all know that bending over a toilet seat with a borrowed tenner, a bag of (mostly) baking powder, and a new best friend isn't a good look at any age, but definitely not post-fifty. If you don't know what I'm talking about, then I applaud your sensible life choices.

That cautionary note aside, midlife is surely no time to turn down substances that genuinely improve your quality of life. In truth, after two years of struggle, I'd have probably embraced an "eye of newt" concoction or something bought on a street corner if someone had told me it would help, but luckily I wasn't mixing in those circles.

When my gynecologist first suggested I try MHT—predominantly to preserve bone density as I edged toward osteoporosis, but also to help with my poor sleep and anxiety—I was only too happy to slap on a patch and to hell with the consequences. At that point, like most women, I thought I knew about the risk MHT might pose when it came to breast cancer, but it seemed worth taking for the sake of a good night's sleep, the end of early-hours anxieties, a boost to my bone and heart health, as well as possibly lowering the chance of type 2 diabetes, various cancers, and—potentially—Alzheimer's disease. I was wary, having suffered from lumps in my breasts (benign and transitory) in the past so I now have regular breast checks.

But I have heard countless stories from across the States (and all too similar tales in the UK) about women being refused or not offered MHT. It's amazing how many opinions there are about what women should and shouldn't do with our bodies, and how much pain we ought to endure, that don't come from women themselves. As delivery vessels for the species, we've been considered common property since time began. Decisions about what is and isn't best for us have, for thousands of years, been made by people with an entirely different perspective, plus a penis. Indeed, in an era of conspiracy theories I have one of my own. It involves a secret cabal giving women unmitigated access to a tsunami of products on the beauty front that promise the impossible, but denying us imperative information and access to things that can change our lives (and even looks—hair, skin, nails, etc.) for the better like MHT.

We now understand that the physiological differences between men and women are far more extensive than simply having different sex organs. The fact that women are governed by estrogen and men by testosterone means that our reactions to many conditions and medications are different. But how can men possibly comprehend specifically female experiences, such as childbirth, pregnancy, periods, and menopause, let alone the need to alleviate any pain or symptoms?

A friend of mine explains the lack of male empathy for female complaints (clearly, this is a massive generalization) by pointing out that her husband was dismissive to the point of rudeness about the agony of childbirth, but incredibly loving whenever she had a hangover. "He understood that pain, so he was able to empathize," she says (incidentally, they are now divorced).

I'm pretty sure that almost every woman of perimenopausal age, regardless of symptoms, has a strong opinion about menopause and most middle-aged men don't. One woman recently told me that her doctor stated that he didn't agree with MHT, so wasn't going to prescribe it for her. According to this medically trained man she could apparently do perfectly well without it. I wonder what study his opinion was based on, or whether he'd just been flicking through his morning newspaper . . . or whether he ever posed himself the same question before taking a painkiller or Viagra, which is available over the counter in the UK.

The MHT 101

While I do occasionally look back to my first, mostly medication-free, four decades, my current reliance on a daily squirt of gel and nightly popping of a pill seems a small price to pay for so many health benefits. It took a few months to find the right cocktail, but it really works for me. As every woman's menopause is different, so you are entitled to a personalized prescription. Although not widely advertised (and why, one wonders, is that, since we represent a huge market) MHT is not a one-size-fits-all scenario. What suits one woman may be catastrophic for another. There are more than fifty variations available: patches, pills, gels, and even implants. How on earth do you know which one you should take?

Do I Need It?

Dr. Minkin says: We try to find out where the patient is on the perimenopause continuum, mostly based on symptomatology. Estrogen is available in two forms: body identical 17-beta-estradiol, derived from plant sources such as yams, and conjugated estrogens, which are older versions made from pregnant mares' urine (Premarin) or other sources.

How Do You Take It

Dr. Minkin says: MHT can be given as oral tablets or transdermal (17-beta-estradiol), which means it's absorbed via the skin and comes as a gel, patch, or spray. The patches are placed on the abdomen or butt (you get higher absorption on the butt!), the gels go on the arms or thighs, and the transdermal spray on the thinner forearm. One of the problems with the gel is that you can't achieve a super high level of estrogen. A couple of groups will unquestionably do better with transdermal estrogen—those who have migraine for example, who are very sensitive to hormonal fluctuation. There's a vaginal ring available for systemic therapy, but this isn't widely used.

If one thing doesn't work, try another, and you can titrate doses until hot flashes improve, you sleep better, and your vagina is more comfortable. You'll know if you're using too much because you'll probably have bloating, aching breasts, and queasiness.

Why Do You Need Progesterone?

Dr. Minkin says: If you have a uterus, you have to keep the womb lining from getting too thick (which increases the risk of endometrial cancer), and so you need a progestogen (a form of progesterone) alongside estrogen. This is called "combined MHT," and can be in the form of a synthetic progestogen (a progestin) or micronized progesterone. Alternatively, the Mirena intrauterine system (IUS) is licensed as contraception. Though not officially prescribed as MHT, if a woman is using it for contraception in perimenopause, it also protects the womb lining, and you take estrogen alongside. This is excellent if women aren't having significant vasomotor symptoms (hot flashes) but are having bleeding.

For women in perimenopause, in good health, not significantly obese, and who are non-smokers, combined hormonal contraceptives can be fabulous for controlling symptoms.

How Long Can I Take MHT?

Dr. Minkin says: The American College of Obstetricians and Gynecologists has issued an official position statement saying that there is no need to stop at the age of sixty or sixty-five.

Mariella says: As I've already announced, I have no intention of stopping, and we've spoken to women in their seventies and eighties who are quite happy with their MHT. When you stop is a joint decision between the patient and her healthcare provider.

What If I Want to Stop?

If you do come off MHT, it doesn't start menopause all over again. You will just reenter it; you might have no symptoms and you might have the same or new ones.

Dr. Minkin says: No literature suggests that tapering is any less problematic than cold turkey, but an experienced menopause doctor will recommend tapering. Practical experience supports this. If someone wants to stop, avoid hotter months—hot flashes will be worse if they do return. Do it gradually in cooler months.

How to Use It

There are two ways of administering combined MHT: cyclical and continuous combined. With continuous combined you take estrogen and a progestogen every day and don't have a bleed. This works best for women who are fully menopausal as opposed to those in perimenopause.

"You can do cyclical therapy in perimenopause: introducing the progestogen for ten to fourteen days a month to produce a cycle with a regular withdrawal bleed," says Dr. Minkin. "Even in a woman who has gone a full year without a period, I often use cyclical because there may be breakthrough bleeding with continuous combined."

Around one in five women is sensitive to progestogen. If you had PMS when younger, then you may find that this is the case, and this can lead to irritability, sore breasts, or spotting. "Some progestogens are better tolerated, such as micronized progesterone. But five percent of women even struggle with this, in which case we have to go to other options, such as the Mirena IUD, or a newer option, bazedoxifene which is a SERM (selective estrogen receptor modulator) and a progesterone-free option."

Do I Need Testosterone?

We used to think that men had a monopoly on testosterone, but it turns out women also rely on smaller levels for energy, libido, and even to boost mood. Some readers may be thinking at this point that their partner needs a top up! There has been something of a gold rush on testosterone in the UK, but in fact it doesn't benefit all women. You need to have your levels checked and then use it for three months to see whether there's any difference. The ovaries continue to produce some testosterone after menopause. There's currently only evidence for its efficacy in libido, but anecdotally many women report other benefits.

Dr. Minkin says: The only official indication is for libido, although it's widely used for energy and building muscle mass. And despite the International Menopause Society and The Menopause Society officially endorsing it for libido, it's not officially approved by the FDA and there's not an FDA-approved product in the States. This means that we have to use the formulations made for men, though in far smaller doses.

(It can be obtained from compounding pharmacies, but because of the lack of official FDA approval, insurers won't cover it for use in women, so they have to pay for it themselves.)

Mariella says: It's much the same situation here in the UK, and I found myself being given tiny tubes of something called Testim, a clear gel replacement testosterone formulated for men that smelled of very cheap aftershave on me, I had to measure it out carefully (a blob the size of a dime). I don't know if my downy chin was a direct result but shortly afterward I embarked on my debut face wax! Now there's a blessedly scent-free cream called Androfeme, out of Australia, that's formulated specifically for women and available in the UK, but it's expensive and only a small group of doctors prescribe it. You may decide you're better off smelling like a teenage boy at his high school prom!

Bioidentical/Body Identical

I think the question I get asked the most is what's the difference between bioidentical and body identical MHT. The days of using pigs' ovaries are thankfully behind us! The most recent types of MHT are described as both body identical and bioidentical and have the same molecular structure as the hormones that we produce in our bodies. This estrogen is derived from yams, in the form known as 17-beta-estradiol, and the progestogen is micronized progesterone, also from plant sources, and available as a tablet.

Now it gets confusing. There are also what's known as bioidentical custom-compounded hormones, and these take the form of personalized prescriptions made in compounding pharmacies.

Experts do not often recommend these, as they haven't been subjected to the same rigorous testing and trials as the regulated products and do not have FDA approval. There is readily available FDA-approved 17-beta-estradiol (identical to that produced by the ovaries) and progesterone (ditto), and these are made in pharmaceutical labs and under FDA supervision.

Dr. Minkin says: Bioidentical is a marketing term, and NOT a medical term. Compounding pharmacies can be excellent for making up unusual doses that aren't made by pharma companies, and for dissolving hormones into different bases—for example, if someone has a peanut allergy and the commercial product is dissolved in a peanut oil base. Compounding pharmacies aren't subject to FDA supervision.

The most important thing to realize is that all FDA approved products must have a package insert with all the potential complications that can happen with a product. Compounding pharmacies do not have these inserts, but the products have exactly the same potential side effects.

(If you don't have very specific needs it's far better to use MHT that has been FDA approved rather than these less reliable formulations, which tend to cost more and have far less research and science behind them.)

Vaginal Estrogen

We cover dry vaginas, so to speak, in chapter ten, but it's worth mentioning vaginal estrogen here. Despite being an essential supplement for women experiencing the drying effects from the loss of estrogen, this is still very much under the radar. It has no cancer risk, and there are plenty of preparations—pessaries, gel, tablets, and creams that are applied locally and are beneficial for the vagina and the bladder, all of which rely on estrogen to stay supple and lubricated. And the good news, you can have systemic MHT and vaginal estrogen at the same time.

Protect the Heart

There's a trio of body parts that are very much supported by MHT—the heart, bones, and brain. Heart disease runs in my family, so this concerns me in a very personal way. According to the CDC, over 60 million women in the United States are living with some form of heart disease, and it's the leading cause of death for women. In 2021, it was responsible for the deaths of 310,661 women.

Women are far more likely to develop coronary heart disease postmenopause. This is a state of affairs only recently recognized. The American Heart Association points out that as women go through menopause our cardiovascular risks rise. We lose the protective factor of estrogen, which helps to control cholesterol levels and reduces the build-up of the plaque that narrows the arteries in a condition known as atherosclerosis, and this means you are more likely to develop coronary heart disease or suffer a stroke.

According to the US Office on Women's Health, women fare worse after heart attacks compared to men, and women are less likely to join and complete a cardiac rehab program. "Heart disease presents differently in women," says cardiologist Dr. Roxana. "We have different plaque characteristics, different fat distribution, and so many different biologies that need taking into account." Should we present with heart attacks, we are, she says, less likely to leave with lifesaving therapies. "This is unconscionable." She adds that we shouldn't be waiting until menopause to make potentially lifesaving lifestyle changes. "Women should be proactive at their healthiest level so when the mask comes off it looks pretty damn good underneath."

Boning Up on the Facts

Those at risk of osteoporosis should also consider the benefits of MHT. Estrogen protects osteoblasts, which are the cells that produce bone. When estrogen levels drop, these aren't able to function effectively and you lose bone density and flexibility. In the five to seven years after menopause, when estrogen production has plummeted, you can lose as much as twenty percent of your bone mass, meaning that you are more likely to suffer fractures.

The Bone Health and Osteoporosis Foundation says that approximately 10 million Americans have osteoporosis and another 44 million have low bone density, placing them at increased risk. Approximately half of women will break a bone because of osteoporosis. There is a strong inherited risk: if your mother has osteoporosis, you are more likely to develop it. MHT can be prescribed as a treatment for osteoporosis, to help stop bone loss and prevent fracture. I was surprised to be asked to be tested for bone density before I went on MHT and even more so to discover I was severely osteopenic, the stage where bones are thinning, and which can lead to full-blown osteoporosis. I started taking MHT and exercising, and within two years my condition was reversed (more on bone density and treatment in chapter six).

Dementia Fears

Dementia is a very real and personal fear for me. My grandmother suffered from it, my mother now has it so badly she is in a care home, and her brother, my uncle, is also deep in its grip. As it is believed to travel down the maternal line, it's a concern for me and also for my children. "Brain fog" affects many of us at this point in our lives, and MHT can help with this, but it is also thought that estrogen is a protective factor against developing Alzheimer's.

There's certainly increasing evidence to suggest this, though—spoiler alert—more research is needed.

In 2023, a meta-analysis of six clinical trials and forty-five observational studies of over 6 million women revealed that those using estrogen-only MHT in midlife to treat menopause symptoms were less likely to develop dementia than those who hadn't. Those taking it age sixty-five and older didn't have this benefit.

"Equally, people need to realize that MHT isn't the panacea," says Dr. Neill Epperson, chair of the Department of Psychiatry at the University of Colorado School of Medicine-Anschutz Medical Campus. "Estrogen treatment helps some people more than others. And that's why it's really important to think about MHT from a personalized medicine standpoint. One's current health, age at menopause, or previous life events may alter the balance between benefits and risk of using MHT. For example, we conducted a study with postmenopausal women who underwent multiple adverse childhood experiences before the age of eighteen. When these women were low on estrogen, their brains responded differently when they were trying to do a working memory task compared to women who had not experienced multiple childhood adversities. But when we gave both groups estrogen back, the activity in that part of the brain was indistinguishable between the two groups.

"It's not just about loss of hormones to the brain," says Dr. Epperson. "It's about multiple factors. While we don't yet have a fountain of youth, there are definitely things we can do better. Moderate exercise, a healthy diet, meditation, and positive time with loved ones help us to combat the stress and hassles of daily living. There is extensive research showing that these health-promoting behaviors are very good for brain health, including mood and cognition. We just have to try to take care of ourselves the best we can."

How—and I think most of us have wondered this at one point or another—do you know whether you have normal brain aging or dementia? "This is a common concern," says Dr. Epperson. "Some people lose their train of thought during a conversation or forget what they were going to do when someone distracts them." She says that this experience is most related to the workings of a part of the brain referred to as the prefrontal cortex. The prefrontal cortex helps us to plan, pay attention, recall names and items quickly, and stay focused and organized. "But if—for example— you grew up making buttermilk biscuits like I did, and you have always been able to make them without a recipe, but then you start forgetting the ingredients and the various steps, this could be a sign of early dementia, which first impacts another part of the brain called the hippocampus. This is when I would see a doctor for a cognitive evaluation."

When MHT Is a Must

Around five percent of women go through early menopause—before age forty-five, and one to three percent go through premature menopause— before age forty. This might be as a result of surgery to remove ovaries, che-motherapy, radiotherapy, or genetics. POI—primary or premature ovarian insufficiency—is when ovaries stop working properly before age forty, in up to ninety percent of cases with no explanation. It's related to problems with follicles; because of genetics, autoimmune or metabolic conditions, toxins or cancer treatments. With POI between five and ten percent of women may ovulate and conceive.

All women need support and most need hormone therapy to protect the heart, brain, and bones up to at least the age of fifty-one (Dr. Minkin points out that the majority of oncologists aren't going to recommend or agree to hormone therapy after breast cancer).

"Post-hysterectomy (including removal of ovaries), women are in a significant menopausal state," says Dr. Minkin. "The recommendation is hormone therapy at least till the age of menopause. When ovaries are left in place, they tend to stop working a year or two earlier than they might have done otherwise."

The Advancing Health After Hysterectomy Foundation (AHAH!) was founded in 2014 by Dr. Philip Sarrel, professor emeritus of obstetrics, gynecology, and reproductive sciences at Yale School of Medicine, to support women who had had a hysterectomy and were therefore able to take estrogen-only hormone therapy. AHAH focuses on the high number of women in the United States who have had a hysterectomy by age sixty. Lack of appropriate advice can mean catastrophic health problems developing in later life.

Conclusion

What's clear from the growing body of evidence that is finally being amassed is that some form of MHT is a vital treatment for most women. Maintaining optimal hormone levels isn't a luxury; it's the ultimate health choice, even a necessity, to keep you fit and strong for the years ahead. The longer you are without estrogen, the more likely you are to suffer from the conditions I've described.

Menopause care is an art, involving evidence-based medicine, good communication and interpersonal relationships with patients, identifying and meeting them at their point of need and supporting them along this journey. There are so many permutations. Every woman is different and this needs to be recognized, but we also need to be less passive in accepting unsubstantiated, and in some cases totally wrong-headed, advice.

There are huge benefits from making MHT your first rather than last port of call, and a vast body of evidence suggesting that if you want to get the most out of it, then don't think of it as the last resort. Women can be bad at looking after themselves, probably because we spend so much time looking after everyone else. When it comes to midlife, it's no longer a choice; it's essential that you take the time for self-care.

There are plenty of alternative treatments available (many of which we cover in subsequent chapters) should you not be able to take MHT or because you don't wish to, or because it doesn't necessarily ease all symptoms. But at the moment women using it are in the minority as a result of scaremongering, bad advice, and ignorance of the benefits. There is definitely a need to ensure that women get clear, accurate messaging around it and are therefore in possession of the knowledge needed to make informed choices.

Looking after your health in middle age is, for far too many women, a lottery dependent on where you live, what you can afford, the culture you come from, and which healthcare provider you happen to see. In a modern, advanced, civilized society, this is not an acceptable state of affairs.

"The more conversation we have, the better off we are"

STACY LONDON, FIFTIES, STYLIST, AUTHOR, AND CAMPAIGNER, NEW YORK

I feel like the more voices we have the louder the pitch becomes.

At the end of 2016 I had spine surgery and then I lost my dad, whom I was so close to. Those two events exacerbated what was already a severe menopause experience. But I didn't know that night sweats, hot flashes, insomnia, joint pain, muscle fatigue, and memory loss were related. I just thought that I was losing my mind. My doctor said, "Oh, it's menopause, you'll get over it." I felt like, OK, I must be overreacting. I even said to my therapist at one point, "I think I have early Alzheimer's," and she was like, "Well . . . this is what happens in menopause."

I felt so isolated and lonely, thinking how can I be the only one experiencing this? There was so much shame around feeling the transformation into somebody I didn't recognize that I found it hard to talk about it with my friends.

It took my own proactivity, digging and research to understand what was happening, and to get a handle on what menopause is—a life transition. It is not a health condition, but it has effects that require attention. Nobody knew that at the time, and nobody was talking about hormones because they were villainized by that 2002 study. In fact, I was told that not only would MHT give me breast cancer, but because my mother had had a stroke and my dad had heart disease I was just asking for problems. It took seven years for me to realize that if I wasn't on hormones I probably wasn't going to get a good night's sleep again.

Now I feel that we need medical research and we should not have to pay for hormones. We need legislative changes and for companies to recognize that people in menopause need care in the same way that we have breastfeeding rooms for people with babies. And we should be serving those who are most marginalized and who are receiving the least amount of help. The more that we dance together as a community, the more conversation we have, and the more conversation we have and the more information we share, the better off we are.

"I worry about dementia"

ANGIE, FORTY-NINE, HOMEMAKER, SAN FRANCISCO

I'm about to turn fifty and am in fairly acceptable health, except I've been overweight for most of my life. My biggest worry is dementia. My mom had it when she was sixty-six and she passed away a decade later. I remember in the lead up to her diagnosis, when I was only in my early thirties, she had growing fogginess and forgetfulness, and the doctor said it was just depression that hits at this time of life. It's very much on my mind as I approach fifty and am on my own meno-pause journey. My sister and I both have the concern—and it triggers anxiety. Of course, we're both forgetting the odd word here and there and wondering is it menopause or is it dementia?

"There's no provision for POI"

LINDSEY HAGGERTY, THIRTY, MEDICAL ASSISTANT, TENNESSEE

I'm the USA networker for the UK's Daisy Network, which supports women with POI (premature ovarian insufficiency), helping to connect those with it. Usually women contact the UK group or get in touch with me via Instagram. As far as I know we're the only group in the States providing information about POI. It's an under-recognized and very underdiagnosed condition, and I speak with many women who aren't given MHT, which is vital up to the age of natural menopause.

I had my first period aged thirteen, and then it stopped. Six months later my mother brought me to my pediatrician and they sent me to Vanderbilt to get tested. The doctors there said I had low estrogen. I was on birth control through high school and college where I had periods for a little but they slowed and had totally stopped by the time I was at college. I started to have symptoms of menopause—really bad hot flashes and night sweats as well as vaginal dryness. When I was twenty-one I went to my OB/GYN and she officially diagnosed me and referred me to an endocrinologist. He took me off birth control and put me on MHT, which I've now been on for nine years, and which resolved my symptoms.

At the time I felt totally lost. I was starting my master's degree, so I wasn't in the headspace to have kids, but being told I probably wouldn't really hit me hard. I wasn't angry, but I felt very hurt, and I questioned a lot of things. I was given a one percent chance of conceiving naturally. The good thing was, being so close to Vanderbilt, I was able to talk to a genetic counselor and they found that I was missing a piece of a chromosome, which is what's causing it. I've come to love what I'm doing—helping other women who are lost and helping to grow the network.

"I'd finished with my period by forty"

WENDY, FORTY-EIGHT, EMT, NEW YORK

I found out that I was perimenopausal after two miscarriages at age thirty-five—they did some blood work and told me that I was against the clock. We'd wanted to wait a while before getting pregnant again, but the doctor said not to. We decided to take a break anyway but then I got spontaneously pregnant and now have an eleven- and a thirteen-year-old. After my youngest, my period was very erratic and I had some enormous clots. It was all over by the time I was forty. I didn't want to take MHT because I feel that we should trust our bodies to do what they need to do. The hot flashes are very real now, waking me up five out of seven nights, and I sometimes find myself opening windows even in the middle of winter.

"I was progesterone intolerant"

CHRISTINA, FIFTY, HOMEMAKER, VERMONT

I was put on estrogen and progesterone, and immediately I got the most horrifying symptoms. Unbelievable clitoral pain, like when you bang your elbow. I couldn't walk, I couldn't wash myself, and I couldn't wear trousers. My migraines went through the roof. I stopped taking MHT entirely and now that I've no hormones in my system my migraines are a lot better. I also chose not to go back on the mini-pill (progesterone-only pill) and for the first time since my teens (minus during pregnancies and a stint with a copper coil) I was not using some form of hormone birth control, and suddenly I had far fewer migraines than I had had since the onset of puberty. It seems far too pronounced a change to be a coincidence.

I limit sugar, because that's a trigger for my migraines, and I use CBD oil, which has helped with stress. Nobody talks about menopause, but when you crack open the door all the details come out. It's not as though it's forbidden, it's more that if you don't say anything the conversation simply doesn't happen.

"Thank goodness for MHT"

MEAGHAN, FIFTY, BRAND STRATEGY AND
TRANSFORMATION DESIGN CONSULTANT, NEW YORK

About a month ago I started feeling so hot. My face would get beet red, and I'd be boiling behind my knees and my back. At night I'd have to change my T-shirts. I remember thinking "I'm so out of shape" and then realizing, wait a minute! I said to my mom, "I'm getting hot in the weirdest ways," and she said, "I think you're having hot flashes, honey." It's so funny, we know what to expect, but when it happens we're surprised. I'd also been noticing that I was really out of shape. I know my body well, and this wasn't typical. So I now have an estrogen patch, which has made an unbelievable difference, and I'm doing strength training and looking at my nutrition.

CHAPTER FIVE

A Literal "Pause"

Let's take a moment.

When the going gets tough, those in the know take a few slow breaths and look deep inside for strength and awareness. The link between mind and body is long recognized by science, as is the fact that, if you look after either one, the other responds positively. It's a relationship we forget at our peril. That's why many women struggling with menopause may find that proven practices such as yoga, mindfulness, and meditation can come in very handy indeed.

I'm the last person to accept the "overwrought" cliché so often thrown at my sex. Therefore the idea that you can inhale your way through meno-pause is one I initially approached with cynicism. It seemed to play to every stereotype of the hysterical woman, as well as that ill-founded philosophy purported by the likes of Freud: that we are nothing but unhinged weak-lings, dominated by our inferior biology.

Nevertheless, a simple yoga breathing technique to quiet the all-night-long chorus in my brain is one of the most helpful tools I've embraced. I inhale for four seconds, hold my breath for seven seconds, and exhale for eight seconds. I've regularly lain awake in the small hours, breathing deep into my abdomen and counting each breath until my frenzied thoughts subside and I can stop panicking about suddenly urgent matters, such as whether or not I gave the dogs their worm medication. There are occasions when it takes so long I lose confidence that I will find respite, but a good eighty percent of the time it works, which makes it worth the effort! When it comes to what I term "raging brain syndrome," a particular issue for those of us with insomniac tendencies, this is top of my list for helping shrug off negative thoughts and shepherd my meandering mind back to stillness.

Calming yourself down may sound horribly head-patting, but if you have fears about menopause and aging, or feel stressed about having symptoms such as hot flashes, then it's likely to create a negative impact on your well-being. That's why the music in horror films starts putting you on edge long before the gory bits begin. *Jaws* without the dum-dum, dum-dum is just a woman swimming, and *The Omen* is a kid with a grumpy face and a serious case of stink eye. Anticipation is everything when it comes to bad news stories, and this becomes a cycle of stress. The more worried you are, the more you become trapped in an expanding dark cave of negative emotion.

"When I think of what anxiety can trigger, I think of the fight-or-flight response," says OB/GYN and midlife health expert Dr. Taniqua Miller. "Yes, it's how we've been able to survive as a species and not be eaten by a saber-toothed tiger. But when we're anxious we release cortisol—the stress hormone. Exposure to high levels of cortisol on a chronic basis can do a lot of damage to the body, like increased fat storage, higher risk of stroke, or heart problems because of higher blood pressure and digestive problems. Cortisol doesn't know that you're stressed because of the menopausal transition. It's just trying to help you survive."

Thankfully we're not just helpless victims of increased anxiety. We have the capacity to harness negative thoughts and therefore control our cortisol levels. There are ways of thinking yourself off the whirring hamster wheel of fast heartbeat and fear, and convincing your mind to shift sideways into a calm, green pasture of happy thoughts.

A Bloody Quick Global Tour

Global experiences of menopause offer an interesting insight into how culture directly affects experience. In the US the prevailing narrative has, until very recently, been predominantly negative and inaccurate. This is doing women no favors at all. "In societies where age is more revered and the older woman is the wiser and better woman, menopausal symptoms are significantly less bothersome," says Dr. Minkin. "The change is liberating, freeing women from anxieties about childbearing and from pain and discomfort related to their reproductive organs. Where older is not perceived in a positive light, as in most Western cultures, symptoms can be far more debilitating."

It's also pretty widely acknowledged that research has only too often investigated the experience of white women, which means our wider understanding is compromised, to say the least. But where investigations have been more inclusive, they reveal staggeringly different attitudes. A 2007 study conducted in Ecuador found that 93.7 percent of middle-aged women perceived menopause as a normal event, and 78.8 percent said that it gave maturity and confidence. In taped interviews in Jordan, 2008, menopause was seen as a positive transition, and a route to wise old age. Then there's the Hadza tribe of Tanzania, whom we referenced in chapter two as a good example of the grandmother hypothesis, where the older women are vital components of society. They are so frequently written about in anthropological studies that I'm surprised they are able to go about their normal lives without being interrupted every five minutes.

My tribe, such as it is, consists of two teenagers, a hardworking husband, assorted relatives, and excellent friends. To each I give different parts of myself, but I can't say I'm regarded as a wise woman by any of them. Useful? Yes, particularly when people want to be picked up from parties at three a.m. or need money for Uber fares. Respected for my wisdom? Not if you read the social media platform formerly known as Twitter after I've published a column!

What's clear is that your culture's attitude toward menopause affects not just your feelings, but also your experience. Obviously, the whole period (or lack of them—that's almost a menopause joke) is also affected by genetics, lifestyle, and—I strongly suspect—luck of the draw.

As far back as 1975, an anthropologist called Marcha Flint noted that different cultures displayed different responses. She surveyed 483 women from the Indian states of Rajasthan and Himachal Pradesh and noticed that most women suffered no symptoms of menopause. At the same time, she realized that once periods stopped, their quality of life improved. Before menopause, women were expected to wear veils and live secluded lives. Postmenopause, they were allowed to leave the women's quarters and publicly mix and joke with men. Might there, it was wondered, be a link?

Later on, a massive 2015 study led by Dr. Minkin asked more than eight thousand men and women how menopause had affected their sex lives.

Here, complaints were pretty much the same from Sweden to the States. But the level of difficulty in dealing with them differed, depending on how those countries viewed the transition.

Even vocabulary affects our perception. A 2012 study explained that the language used around menopause can demonstrate how a society considers a topic. "Menopause in the Western world is largely medicalized, with much of the language being dominated by negative imagery such as 'reproductive failure' or 'ovarian failure,'" the authors wrote. Clearly, the wording isn't designed to deliberately make you feel bad, but it's not exactly vibrating with positivity. "In the Arab world," it continues, "the word corresponding to the menopausal and mid-life period means 'desperate age.'"

So, if you live in a place where menopause is ignored or seen as a bad thing, it's going to make you feel worse about it. Unless you're given positive imagery and a sense of future advantages, it's no wonder that so many of us approach it with the dread steps of the condemned! How much better would our experience be if it was bathed in a positive light? If our communities at home and at work were seeking us out for wise counsel and revering our longevity, instead of sniggering and going back to their mobile phones because you're just so, like, old.

To be honest, taking control of our thoughts and finding ways to lighten anxiety aren't just skills for menopause, they are skills for life. Our response to danger is what has kept the human race alive, but now that the woolly mammoths are all gone, much of our sense of peril is self-created. Our negative thoughts can become—metaphorically speaking—the saber-toothed tigers of the twenty-first century. If any of this makes you think "Aha! It *is* all in your mind, love," then we've failed in our task. You can't "cure" menopause by controlled breathing, or reaching an elevated state of tranquillity, but every little bit helps. Mind over matter isn't a new concept, but it's one worth investigating and, perhaps, rewording. Mind with matter is the ultimate collaboration, and one I consider well worth aspiring to achieve.

Start with CBT

MHT is not the only way of treating menopausal symptoms, nor is it a wonder drug that alleviates every condition. To support it, and for those who don't wish to or can't take it, there are other therapies that can help to negate the more debilitating impacts of hormone discord.

As I've said, thinking or breathing your way through the unavoidable ebbing of hormones was something I didn't want to believe possible. To say I was extremely skeptical before I made my 2018 menopause documentary is an understatement. But in the show, we conducted a trial with five women who weren't able to take MHT and who all suffered from debilitating hot flashes, with devastating consequences on their quality of life. I watched them go through a four-week program of cognitive behavioral therapy, or CBT, a type of talk therapy, at the end of which they had seen a sixty-four percent reduction in hot flashes, and a ninety-five percent decrease in the night sweats. I sped from skeptic to full fangirl. The transformation in this group of hitherto suffering women was extraordinary; they radiated contentment and confidence.

This was all thanks to the work done by Myra Hunter, emeritus professor of clinical health psychology at King's College London, and the co-author, along with Dr. Melanie Smith, of *Living Well Through the Menopause*. Professor Hunter has devoted her career to exploring the possible links between what we think and how we feel physically, and is frustrated by the fact that, in our culture, everything is attributed to menopause at this time of life. "It means that much of the information available—and especially online—are the extremes, so women unwittingly expect to have all the symptoms, enter this phase with dread, and are therefore more likely to have a negative experience.

"Remember that all pain or physical discomfort is to some extent affected by psychosocial factors." By this, she means that, for example, should you experience chest pain, you'll instantly assume you're having a heart attack because that's what we've been led to believe. I can empathize with this; so much as a twinge in my rib cage, and I'm sitting up in bed wondering whether to poke my husband awake so he can call 911, or suffer quietly, alone, grumpy, and, not to be overly dramatic, possibly dying, although so far that's not happened.

"Eighty percent of people who seek medical advice with chest pain don't have heart problems," says Professor Hunter. "Your reaction to chest pain will also be a stress reaction. This applies to menopause, where symptoms can become a negative cycle. Bear in mind that these are also affected by the ageist and sexist views to which we're exposed."

CBT is helpful for managing hot flashes and quality of life, and mindfulness and yoga are useful for general well-being, she tells me. CBT is effectively a non-medical therapy that helps people to develop practical ways of managing problems and offers coping solutions. The 2023 Menopause Society non-hormone therapy position statement says that "the body of literature as a whole supports that CBT alleviates bothersome VMS (hot flashes) for both survivors of breast cancer and menopausal women." Another nonmedication recommendation is clinical hypnotherapy, which also has solid evidence for reducing hot flashes.

What I love (now) about this approach is that it's cheap and fairly simple. So if you are anxious and stressed, you are encouraged to write down your thoughts, feelings, and reactions and then consider whether they are overly negative. Look at your lifestyle; try to eat and drink sensibly, don't overwork, and (in today's smartphone-induced isolation) don't avoid people.

Professor Hunter says that if you're suffering a hot flash and worry about what people are thinking or noticing, it may make you feel self-conscious, impact your confidence, and intensify the feeling of the flash. "If you are hot and sweating in a meeting, you may think everyone has noticed, and believes you're over the hill." So true—those five women told me that they lived in a state of embarrassment. The flashes felt like an admission that they were getting old.

It wasn't a magic wand that banished symptoms, the participants in the study had to put in some effort. There were interactive sessions and they were asked to put their thoughts and goals in a diary. They were reminded that even relatively small things can make a difference: improvements in well-being, such as reading a book before bed. I know this sounds patronizing; we've all read the women's magazines with listicles of "how to have me-time," and rolled our eyes at the seemingly lazy repetitions of "leave your phone downstairs" and "have a warm bath." But annoyingly condescending as they may seem, like all clichés, they carry some truth.

"The women were also taught paced breathing, an exercise which involves slow, deep breathing from the stomach. The idea is that it may ease anxiety enough to alleviate the hot flash, or even stop it from being fully triggered," says Professor Hunter.

If you don't panic, or get angry and frustrated (easy to say, I know; my temper goes from zero to ten in a heartbeat since menopause), and simply surf the rising heat in your body, then the flashes won't impact your life so much. As I say, the results were quite extraordinary, and because of the interactive nature of CBT, it has the added advantage of being something you have personally achieved, lending a much-needed sense of control over what's happening to your body. It is true empowerment.

Yelling Out for Yoga

Yoga is my other weapon against postmenopause insomnia, stress, and generally seizing up. A handful of times in the last five years, I've gone to a retreat called Yeotown in Devon in the wild (south)west of the UK. Here for five days, I walk, detox (no caffeine, no alcohol, no sugar), and do incredible yoga twice a day with the co-owner and career yogi Mercedes Sieff. If you check her out on Instagram (bearing in mind she's in our menopausal age group) you'll see what our bodies are capable of doing if we put in the hard labor! Obviously, the Yeotown lifestyle is one I aspire to wholeheartedly, but unfortunately, I appear to be very easily distracted from that utopian model the moment I'm not under supervision!

Watching Mercedes lead the first class invariably makes me feel like a calcified toxin-riddled disgrace. Nevertheless, after the program (like rehab!), I always return refreshed, revitalized, and determined to carry on with the good work, until someone plonks a steak and a glass of red wine in front of me and I embrace retoxing with gusto. That's where learning not to load up on guilt comes in very handy. The road to hell, as they say, is paved with good intentions! When I'm low on energy, feeling peaky or overstressed, remembering the lessons from Yeotown helps me to reset. It's a glimpse of how much better we'd all feel without a full-time job, stress, kids, partner, commute, and a dependence on refined carbs to boost energy levels rather than those "powerball" dried fruit–filled alternatives.

Obviously, a few days at a luxury yoga camp is an enormous and expensive treat. When there's a chef concocting glorious gourmet vegan food, it's easy to fantasize that you'll eat like that every day when you're isolated from normal temptations. On a day-to-day basis, managing to resolve life's challenges by eating like a Michelin-starred yogi and summoning up relaxation techniques is an unreachable goal, and we know that setting the bar so high that failure is all but guaranteed does nobody's mental health any favors. But being reminded how good it's possible to feel is a great memory to carry with you. More realistically I still try to do yoga a couple of times a week, but ironically the days when I most need it are those during which I can't even find the time to make the bed before scooting out of the house. However, there's firm evidence and countless positive clinical studies highlighting the benefits of regular yoga for midlife health, and once you know what to do you don't even have to leave your bedroom! It absolutely doesn't have to take place in five-star surroundings.

The physical postures and breathing exercises improve muscle strength, flexibility, blood circulation, and hormone function and the relaxation is beneficial for the brain. There are also specific menopause benefits: yoga helps you to manage stress, anxiety, and insomnia—all boxes I've regularly ticked on the symptom chart.

Yoga fans seem relaxed about the fact that you can call a class anything you like; there is anti-gravity yoga, where you hang upside down; laughter yoga (self-explanatory); and even dog yoga, where you writhe around your bemused hound. In that lineup, menopause yoga sounds positively pedestrian.

"Yoga can be incredibly beneficial both mentally and physically for the perimenopausal and menopausal phase of life, which I like to call the Queen Stage," says New York yoga teacher and yoga therapist Juliana Mitchell. "The practice forces us to befriend transformation, opening the door to seeing the beauty and wisdom in the process rather than the idea of getting older being an enemy. In yoga, traditionally, there's reverence for aging.

"In this transitional stage of life, our hormones are in significant flux. Being in an optimal health state (of mind and body) will create a better scenario for our hormones and thereby for our felt and lived experience. One of the physical forms I teach is restorative yoga, a restful form which is shown to reduce the severity, frequency, and duration of hot flashes. Of the many things it's doing, it reminds the nervous system how to relax deeply, which helps to balance hormones and reduce inflammation, whereas active postures can help maintain bone density and muscle strength." She says that yoga can also help with sleep. "Because of my long-time practice, I am experienced in working with my mind, body, and breath, so I'm able to relax myself if I can't sleep. And I have cooling breaths I can work with if I have hot flashes."

There is also fascinating research showing that when women are stressed, we release oxytocin and seek the company of other women. I can absolutely concur with that, whether I'm doing a downward dog at the same time or not.

Making Time for Meditation

To say I'm not a natural candidate for meditation is a massive understatement. Although I would probably benefit hugely from mastering something that puts boundaries around my brain's restless meanderings, on the few occasions I've tried it, my inability to sit still trumps my higher ambitions. It remains an incentive to master though, because on the few occasions I've gotten close to "freeing" my mind, I've felt infinitely calmer for the effort. My thoughts are far too good at wandering off to deadlines and life logistics, or what Netflix option I'll go for that night. I know that it's a potent therapy, but I'm also aware that I need more discipline!

"There are many forms of meditation," says Dr. Jill Wener, a physician, EFT/tapping practitioner, anti-racism educator, trauma specialist, and certified meditation teacher. "The meditation I teach is about achieving a transcendental state (neither asleep nor awake), and is a way of positively changing how you feel, whether that's being more present in the moment, being more relaxed and less stressed, being more intuitive or healthier." All of which sound positively aspirational to me!

Meditation calms your sympathetic nervous system—deactivating the fight-or-flight response that we've discussed, and it's clinically proven to help with stress. The more you practice it, the calmer you are likely to feel. In terms of menopause, therefore, meditation can benefit many symptoms. "I feel that meditation can also mitigate some of the emotional response, such as any fear or frustration that women are experiencing," says Dr. Wener.

A 2020 study showed that women who meditated at least once a week for six months both eased menopausal symptoms, including a reduction in depression and irritability, and also changed their blood chemistry for the better, suggesting it might help lower risk for cardiovascular disease, and there's some evidence that it might even help with hot flashes.

"There isn't one way to do it," says Dr. Wener. "The way that I teach is using a mantra and very little effort, but there's sound meditation, walking meditation, a top to toe body scan, guided meditations . . . All of these can be beneficial." (Friends highly recommend the Calm, Headspace, and Waking Up apps.)

Mindfulness

Mindfulness, which has enjoyed a huge surge in popularity in recent years, is a form of meditation.

But what is mindfulness? I've always vaguely thought of it as being an appreciation of birdsong, and in fact I'm not a million miles away. Vidyamala Burch, expert, author of *Mindfulness for Women* and co-founder of a Breathworks program, clarifies:

"At its most simple, mindfulness is awareness of what's happening in any moment, whether mentally, physically, or emotionally," she says. "Once we know what we are experiencing in an immediate and direct way, we can then choose how to respond and live with more clarity and confidence. When we are not aware, it's as if we're existing in fog, a self-generated cloud of thoughts and feelings, worries and anxieties, that affect our judgment and so often undermine our mood and even torment us. Mindfulness helps dissolve this fog, so we can 'come home' to our direct experience in any moment—what we see, smell, taste, hear, and touch. We feel more vividly alive as we experience what is actually happening, rather than being lost in all our interpretations, fears, and so on."

This makes infinite sense, and tallies with what I understand as the simplest explanation of mindfulness: that it's appreciation of the moment. Try to experience every moment for what it is, rather than what you project onto it with negative thinking. If you stop and listen to the natural world, you can find your place in it so much improved. See and feel the beauty in the moment. And before you think I've floated off on a cloud of MHT-induced hysteria . . .

"I'm not saying practice this and have an amazing life," Vidyamala says. "There are always difficult things, but awareness builds resilience. The fear of what might happen falls away and you appreciate the present. Everything is pared back to what is happening now, and then the present moment blooms into richness."

To put it even more simply, it's mind training. "We understand physical health and fitness: going to the gym and eating five pieces of fruit and vegetables a day. But there's no decent messaging about our mental health. What makes more sense than training your mind to work with you rather than against you? Training your mind with mindfulness or meditation can become as embedded in your daily routine as flossing your teeth."

As an example of how it might work with menopause, she says that if you are panicking about having a hot flash and worrying about how you feel and how others are looking at you, mindfulness can bring clarity and calm. This is very much in tune with the CBT approach, which employs similar techniques.

The other bonus of meditation and mindfulness is that they're free to practice and you can do a meditation in just one minute, although longer is preferable. You can do it anywhere, although a peaceful location is more conducive to success! And the more you practice, the better you become at staying in the moment and the greater the benefits.

"Mindfulness can have rapid results, and with practice you can radiate calmness, which positively affects those around you," Vidyamala tells me soothingly. Anyone who has met me will know that my natural default is slightly frenetic, my ADHD doesn't help, and my natural resting place is when I'm trying to do ten things at once, but I am charmed by the idea of radiating postmenopausal tranquility.

Three-Minute Meditation by Vidyamala Burch

Sit or lie comfortably and relax. You can be inside or outside. Observe how your body feels: what physical sensations you're experiencing. Is there a cushion behind your back or underneath you? Simply notice the sensations for a few seconds. Now listen to any sounds: loud, soft, high, low. How do you respond to them? Don't try to identify where they're coming from, but just listen. Allow the sounds to come toward you and allow them to flow around you. If it's silent, notice this.

How does your breath feel? What parts of your body are moving as you breathe? Try to be aware of these movements and the sensations of breathing from the inside, rather than as an onlooker. Now move to your emotions. Are you generally happy, sad, calm, or angry? Gently tune into your "emotional weather" without harsh judgment. Can you have a bit of perspective on whatever you're feeling as you quietly sit with the experience of breathing?

Be aware of whatever thoughts are flowing through your mind. See if you can have perspective here, too—let your thoughts be like clouds passing across the blue sky of awareness rather than statements of fact. Can you look at your thoughts rather than from them?

Finally, just rest in your body—be present in the moment and notice breathing, feeling, sounds, and emotions as they happen. Let everything come and go with a sense of flow, moment by moment.

Breathe Deep

Calm breathing tells the body that all is well, even if it's not. It soothes stress and anxiety and boosts the immune system. There is so much evidence about the positive benefits of breathing correctly that people have written entire books about it. This has been the cause of great hilarity in my house, with teenagers hooting with glee at the idea of grown-ups being "so dumb" (not my words, obviously) that they can't even breathe properly.

Breathing Exercise by Vidyamala Burch

Do this whenever you feel it might be helpful.

Feel your feet on the floor and your bottom on the chair, if you're sitting.

Take a deep breath in, bringing your awareness into your abdomen and letting it swell out.

Let the out-breath flow all the way out, letting your abdomen subside back and giving the weight of your body up to gravity, so that it's supported by the floor.

Let the in-breath flow back in again in its own time.

If you can, let this embodied breath awareness be an anchor for the mind as you keep giving your weight up to the support of gravity with each out-breath. Allow your thoughts to come and go like clouds in the sky.

Tapping

I'm afraid I've always been rather dismissive about tapping. How can gently hitting parts of your own body whilst talking to yourself alleviate stress? It seems to me that it's a sort of self-care that is guaranteed to send me into a flat spin and double my stress levels. But Dr. Wener says that tapping is like magic. "It's loosely based on traditional Chinese medicine and stimulates acupressure points around the face and upper body to unblock the flow of energy through the body." Tapping, or EFT—emotional freedom technique—was developed by a psychologist in the 1980s and refined and made popular in the 1990s. "Tapping is like spot cleaning," she says. "It doesn't need to be done in a therapeutic environment. What I love is that it's a way for people to lean into uncomfortable emotions that we're told to push away, and it can be used in a million ways." There is some good evidence for tapping and menopause symptoms: a 2021 study concluded that tapping for eight weeks significantly reduced the mean score for depression in postmenopausal women.

There are nine main tapping points: the eyebrow, side of the eye, under the eye, under the nose, chin, collarbone, under the arm, top of the head, and side of the hand. Each of these corresponds to a meridian, as per Chinese medicine, and are basically energy pathways through the body.

"By tapping on each of these points and saying what concerns you out loud, the parasympathetic nervous system is activated, and our neural pathways rewired," Dr. Wener explains. It's thought that the physical action of tapping interrupts the fight-or-flight response and also increases endorphins. So in terms of peri- or menopause, it can be used for symptoms such as hot flashes, brain fog, anxiety, stress, and insomnia.

I remain unconvinced that simply telling myself I'm not stressed is going to bring me down from the ceiling, but she says that the best way to tap is to have a specific feeling or problem, and directs me to her YouTube channel so I can do a tapping session for irritability. First, I check in with my irritability to see how strong it is—I give it a nine out of ten. Then I sense where it's present—I can feel knots of ill-humor in my chest and my arms—and start tapping repetitively and a few times each on the top of my head, the side of my eye, under my eye, under my nose, my chin, my collarbone, and under my arm, whilst saying to myself how very irritable I am, why I'm irritable (work stress), and why it's valid. After two rounds of this I check in with myself. The irritability is still there, but slightly less. I do it twice more, acknowledging my irritability once again (and feeling a little silly). It is almost with reluctance that I admit I feel far more relaxed and that the irritability is much diminished. Worth a go, everybody! It really is magic!

Conclusion

As a committed stress-bag, I know it seems unlikely that stepping off the regular treadmill of your existence for five minutes a day will have a beneficial impact. Yet the most important thing I've learned on my own adventure is to remember that we have (only) one body, one mind, and one life. I can't help wondering whether menopause is also a reminder to women, who carry so much of the world on their shoulders, that we are not invincible. We need to stop trying to take care of everyone around us and try to take better care of ourselves. There is no harm in discovering how best you can press the pause button and breathe new life into your body.

Namaste!

"Take stock of your life and where you want to go."

STACY LONDON, FIFTIES, STYLIST, AUTHOR,
AND CAMPAIGNER, NEW YORK

Menopause is a moment of reckoning. I don't mean to give that a negative connotation. You've been with your partner for however long, you have empty nest syndrome, you're dealing with elder care, you're under a lot of financial pressure, just when people say you've tapped out in terms of the job market . . . What I mean is, it's a time when you have to sit back and take deep stock of your life and where you want to go.

"I'm learning to be friends with aging"

NADIA NARAIN, FIFTIES, YOGA AND BREATHWORK TEACHER, LOS ANGELES AND LONDON

I used to use yoga as my only form of exercise, but now I do weights and walking, and use yoga more for stress, mobility, and because I love it.

It's important to accept that there might be a change to what you've been doing with yoga, as our bodies go through menopause and a hormonal shift—it's like becoming a mother or a teenager.

Personally, stress takes my symptoms to another level. When I manage my stress, my symptoms are so much better—no hot flashes and I sleep well.

I feel I grew up with women around me who had such a fear of aging. You could never ask a woman her age, and the focus was always about looking younger than they were.

Well, I'd like to do things differently, although it's not easy. Do I look in the mirror and say, "Oh my God, I could probably use a facelift or something"? Sometimes! It's a shock on certain days. But I do try to be more accepting of aging. It's happening whether I like it or not. So maybe acceptance, kindness, and self-love are a few good ingredients.

I'm inspired when I see women confidently gray and confident with their age. I haven't totally let my hair go gray, but I think about it a lot. I feel like I'm the most honest I've ever been with myself and I hope to inspire rather than be afraid.

"I thought I had dementia"

PATSY KENSIT, FIFTIES, ACTOR, LONDON

Nothing prepared me for menopause. Aged forty-five, I was whisked into the hospital for an emergency hysterectomy. I was in the ICU for two days, and we discovered that I didn't have ovarian cancer, which was a huge relief. However, I fell instantly into full menopause.

I started to get terrible brain fog, which developed into anxiety. I had hot flashes, a dry mouth, and couldn't sleep. Someone unhelpfully pointed out that I had developed a slight stutter, and I once found myself in the supermarket completely unaware of why I'd gone in, and I left with a cabbage and a pair of tights. I'd driven since the age of seventeen, and I couldn't drive. I honestly thought I might have dementia: my train of thought would just go, mid-conversation.

My lowest menopausal moment was also my most public. The hospital had given me MHT in the form of patches and creams, but I didn't feel it was working for me, so I was persuaded to try an MHT implant. The next day, I went on a morning talk show. I knew I was feeling terrible, and apologized; the implant had triggered a migraine, which made me so ill I was barely able to speak. In retrospect, I ought to have said that I was sick and left. But I'm a professional, and I soldiered on.

What happened next was shocking. After stumbling through the interview, I was widely accused of being drunk or on drugs. It was such a public moment, and I was devastated. I pride myself on my clarity. A few weeks later, I went back on the show to explain fully, and lots of people called in with their stories. Eventually, I said, "Stop talking about my womb, get on with the show, and I'm off to have a hot flash!"

"It's a holistic process"

BECKS, FORTY-SIX, INTERIOR DESIGNER, CALIFORNIA

It's so wild that menopause isn't discussed. If it's mentioned, everyone wants to share information, but it's not often the subject is brought up. I was getting all zesty and angry a couple of years ago and having big mood swings. I went to my OB/GYN and she put me on the synthetic pill to manage my symptoms. But I didn't like this—it gave me a heavy period and I didn't feel that it was dealing with the problem, so I saw a new doctor and she said that we could manage with diet and supplements and gave me a protocol that included supplements, natural progesterone cream that I put on my wrist, and some Female Balance drops that I put under my tongue twice a day. When I use the cream it stops my hot flashes and I sleep soundly. But the mood swings aren't yet under control and I've been having a lot of anxiety. I firmly believe that it's about looking at the whole picture; diet and exercise as well as hormone levels.

"The US is like a lot of different countries"

BETHANY, FORTY-FIVE, BRAND CONSULTANT, OREGON

I don't think people realize that America is a bunch of different cultures. Someone in Seattle, Washington, will be totally different from someone in Tulsa, Oklahoma. Even in, say, Texas, the cities tend toward the democratic, but everything changes in the rural areas. That means there's still stigma about having menopause treatment in different places, and the benefits versus risks haven't yet filtered down regarding treatments. MHT is still stigmatized and there's not always access to it. We base a lot of information on old research that we've allowed to become law in our minds.

CHAPTER SIX

Meno a-Go-Go

At the age of fifty-two, I took up regular running. Until then, I'd describe myself as having remained base-level fit. I reached that depressing moment in my thirties when getting exercise became necessary, rather than something I occasionally enjoyed. Walking—a love of trekking and pounding paths in the great outdoors—had always been my therapy. But in my thirties I supplemented this with going to the gym (the potential dating pool there was valuable in pre-internet-hook-up days!), and in my forties I realized that I needed to stretch out my compacting skeleton, and found yoga, which, along with daily dog-walking, seemed perfectly adequate. Now, in my early sixties, I am probably the fittest I've ever been—one of the benefits of having grown-up children is that there's more time for exercise, which is now both my hobby and my luxury. How times have changed!

I say exercise is my luxury but when you reach midlife and beyond it's a compulsory duty if you want to live well through your second phase of life. Whatever life stage you're at, diet and exercise choices have an impact on how you feel physically and emotionally, as well as providing a template for future health. When it comes to menopause, the fitter you are and the more you embrace healthy habits, the easier the transition is likely to be.

Mine may sound like a substantial commitment to fitness, but honestly it was low-level mitigation for a lifestyle that was otherwise stress-dominated, reliant on alcohol to relax, and punctuated by irregular meals based on convenient foodstuffs rather than nutritional value. Truthfully, my small-scale exercise regime had a lot to compete with on the retoxing front. But it worked for decades. I was slim, reasonably energetic, and seemingly silver bullet (the tequila-based cocktail) proof.

When I hit fifty, I hit a wall. A hangover would snake painfully around my head for twenty-four hours or more, and I started selecting nights I could let my hair down based on days when I wouldn't be working. It wasn't that I was drinking more, but the recovery period seemed to have doubled. The expectation of a late night also became a new consideration in my diary. I've never been a great sleeper, but now I was tossing and turning all night with palpitations and anxiety, yet lucky to wake up any later than six a.m. That made the clock ticking anywhere close to midnight a Cinderella-style cut-off point for social activity.

Wondering why my body appeared to be failing, I did some research. The rather grim reading contained certain inevitabilities about women developing higher body fat, lower bone density, declining muscle, and an increasing physical inability to process alcohol, all of which are related to those pillars of passing time: menopause and the natural process of aging.

I realized that this was a time to be treated as a challenge, a mountain to be climbed. The only intelligent option was for me to face the fact that, like a boxer heading for a prize fight, aiming for peak health and fitness was going to be necessary for my future. Sitting back and passively accepting decline would, I suspected, swiftly become a self-fulfilling prophecy.

To my dismay, feeling exhausted by plentiful new challenges that seemed to be presenting themselves, I discovered that lethargy can, quite genuinely, cause premature death. Prolonged sedentary behavior in adulthood increases the risk of cardiovascular disease, type 2 diabetes, and some cancers and is directly related to earlier mortality. Appealing though it may seem, your fifties is not the time to slump onto a fireside chair and relax gently into your supposed "twilight" years, unless you want the sun to set on your life a lot earlier than necessary!

Clearly, it was time to galvanize myself. With a bit of knowledge and will-power, we can nurture our bodies and minds for the future, which is more likely to be long and filled with new adventures if you make a few lifestyle changes.

I realized that what I'd taken for granted for decades in terms of health and fitness had now become an essential life goal. As much as we need to prepare ourselves mentally, rejecting the mythology that's kept us ignorant and afraid, we also need to counteract and balance what's happening physically in order to battle the detrimental impact of declining hormones.

I firmly advocate taking this as a "knowledge is power" situation. Let's rise above the doom, and be grateful for the evidence confirming that, if we acknowledge the years around menopause as being a time to amend our ingrained habits, embrace exercise, eat more fiber but less sugar, and consume less booze, we can set ourselves on a path to a more energetic and healthier future.

Don't bury your head in the sand. Confront your past choices and learn your family history, know your blood pressure and your blood sugar and cholesterol levels. Do what you can to boost your chances of a postmenopausal half century in the best possible health. Toast yourself with a small vodka and soda, the least brutal of poisons in my opinion, and bear in mind that it's never too late to make changes, whether you're in your thirties, forties, or your nineties!

Gravity, having children, and years in sedentary jobs will inevitably take their toll. Whether to get your gloves off is a personal choice. My rallying call is to understand what's happening, take control and determine to surf the waves, large and small with as much skill, expertise, and style as can be mustered.

Basically, it's a good time to pick up the mantle of Dylan Thomas and "Rage, rage against the dying of the light." Although, in this case, the "light" is our natural youthful energy, our lean body mass, and our fast metabolism, rather than the grim reaper herself.

The Hangover Equation: It's Time to Talk About Alcohol

$$\frac{\text{Dehydration} \times \text{Age}}{\text{Stress}} = \text{Sleeplessness} + \text{2-day headache}$$

Speaking as someone who once spent four days holed up at the Hotel du Cap during the Cannes Film Festival with a selection of debauched movie moguls and George Clooney, with barely an afternoon nap as sustenance, then went straight to work on Monday morning—you can appreciate that imbibing is an activity of which I have some experience.

Now those happy decades when any problem could be diminished by a vat of fermented grape juice are well and truly behind me. Most women approaching their fifth decade and beyond will vividly recall the downsides of the fun: the horror of waking in the early hours and praying you didn't slur your words. Sleepless nights, miserable moods, bags under your eyes, and puffy skin are all the enemies of elegant aging.

The worsening hangovers are linked to age and hormones, yes, but also connected with levels of hydration, stress, and sleep quality. Looking forward to arid, alcohol-free decades is enough to make any woman reach for the Chardonnay, but the truth is, it's time to cut down on the quaffing.

Does that mean that we have to become teetotalers? Not necessarily. There are ways around this. My co-author, Alice, a lifelong dry white wine drinker—has found herself increasingly drawn to light and fizzy rosé wine with a lower alcohol percentage.

I like the "no drinking at home" rule, which guarantees most of us at least half the week giving our livers time off. Advanced non-drinkers will be able to graduate to "not drinking during the week," though this can create a detox/retox mentality and terrible Sunday-night demons. Science is pretty clear that binge drinking can be as bad as daily drinking.

For all the many downsides, I refuse to give up alcohol completely. I'll tell you why. When I get home from a week in London on a Friday night, the house is usually chaotic. The children's school uniform, or whatever they've been wearing, is laid out on assorted floors, like so many murdered bodies, as is an accumulated heap of wet towels. The dishwasher is full and dirty and chances of supper are 50/50, as my husband and I share the cooking when we're both around. This is clearly a highly frustrating state of affairs. But one lovely glass of red wine or a long, cool Skinny Bitch cocktail (composed of vodka, lime juice, and soda water), and I see my family in a far more benign light. They become charmingly bohemian rather than slovenly and irritating pigs.

Make Your Choice—Wine or Whine

I recall being told that the way in which alcohol guidelines were decided was entirely arbitrary—although perhaps that was what I wanted to believe back in the hedonistic days when I didn't count how many drinks I was consuming. But it's certainly a fact that the recommended amount seems to be getting lower every year. In 1979, in the UK, the official drinking advice was no more than 56 units (one unit = 10ml or 8g of pure alcohol) a week for men—that's around 5½ bottles of wine. To paraphrase Bob Dylan, the times are certainly changing! In the US, it's recommended that women of legal drinking age consume no more than one drink or less per day. The new recommendations in Canada are—to give you a sense of proportion—two standard drinks or less per week. In the UK, hedonists that we are, it's currently no more than 14 units a week, spread across three days or more—about a bottle and a half of wine. It's sobering stuff.

"Alcohol is essentially a poison that your body has to break down and eliminate," says registered holistic nutritional consultant Alyssa Flegg. There are, she says, two main problems with alcohol consumption. "By the time you get to menopause, your liver has probably already been subjected to a fair amount of abuse, working hard to process everything we consume, from nutrients to medications. Many of us will have lost a little liver function or could have the beginnings of fatty liver." It's the aging process rather than menopause that means alcohol is processed more slowly in the body, especially the female body (we often contain less water and more fat), but as we struggle through perimenopause, estrogen can actually be as much as three times higher, and that excess also has to be processed via that poor overworked organ.

The bad news for those who like an evening cocktail is that alcohol can be directly linked to menopause symptoms. "Both alcohol and caffeine could be triggers for hot flashes and night sweats," says Alyssa. In fact, women who drink every day are more likely to suffer from these. Interestingly, she says that different drinks have different impacts—red wine is worse than whisky, though this appears to be anecdotal. I suspect it would be hard to get the funding for a clinical study, though I wouldn't mind taking part in that one! "Many women struggle to sleep during menopause, and alcohol has a terrible effect on sleep." It also has a detrimental effect on mood; if you're feeling low, the worst thing you can do is drink through the dark emotions.

To add to this litany of doom, alcohol has links to all manner of other conditions, such as an increased risk of many cancers, including breast cancer, as well as heart disease, liver disease, and stroke, and it affects the brain. It's also linked to weight gain; in addition to containing empty calories, it increases hunger, makes us crave greasy, salty food, and then stops the body from burning fat because we're too busy trying to metabolize the booze.

This doesn't mean we all need to turn to total abstinence, though some of the above facts might well put you off. "I don't necessarily recommend giving up completely," says Alyssa. "It's a personal decision for everyone. Consider why you're having a drink and try to consume alcohol earlier in the evening so that it doesn't disrupt sleep as much." There are studies showing the benefits of consuming alcohol (in moderate amounts) in the company of friends, so don't feel you have to dismiss it entirely.

Weighty Matters

Ultra-processed food = Weight gain
Slower metabolism

Like most women, my weight has always been irrevocably tied to my mental state. But that stops being an option as metabolism slows down. None of us can rely on meeting a new partner or getting a new job and instantly dropping ten pounds.

It is a cruel time of life, when the woman versus weight-gain battle steps up a notch for us all. I struggled with yo-yoing weight in my early twenties, linked almost entirely to my turbulent emotional life. Happy and in love, I'd become waif thin. Depressed and alone, I could gain several pounds in a matter of weeks. The real benefit of youth is how swiftly the impact of bad living can be negated. By your fifties, the ability to bounce back from bad lifestyle choices is not something you can rely on. As with puberty, we're back on an emotional roller coaster, but fallbacks like comfort eating, slumping in defeat, and dodging the world (as teenagers are wont to do) are no longer options.

For decades, my diet kept me in a fluctuating but tolerable personal weight range. But then, in my early fifties, I began to pile on the pounds, particularly around my tummy, while my thighs became a road map of dimples. Having not really worried about my body or my health since my thirties (during my twenties I worried about everything), now I started to wonder if this was the beginning of the road to oblivion, and, truth be told, it felt a little premature.

It's tricky, because I have no time to bother with the majority of diets out there. From keto to cabbage soup, to maple syrup or apple cider vinegar, anything that involves elaborate menus, significant effort, or questionable science isn't for me. They also subscribe to a societal assumption that thin is aspirational whereas the focus for all of us should be on health, not dress size.

I've learned that sugar in any guise is not my friend, and that it takes determination and commitment to compensate for unpleasant and sudden physical surprises, such as the inability to drop four pounds in as many days to fit into a favored outfit! Food in midlife should be thought of as fuel and like any engine you'll perform better on the right variety. We do need to eat in order to stay alive, so that's a bit of good news! Even if you're lying in bed all day, three quarters of your energy requirement is being used up just keeping your heart beating, your lungs working, and your brain thinking. Sadly, this doesn't mean you can eat minimally, stay in bed, and consider yourself an athlete. I'm sure I'm not the only woman with a recurring fantasy about lying horizontal and doing absolutely nothing for days, but funnily enough, this is not what any experts recommend.

All this said, we need to stop obsessing about being a few pounds lighter. Healthy, strong, happy, and (reasonably) fit is far more important than being size zero.

Stave Away the Surplus

The 2020–2025 dietary guidelines for Americans (we read this stuff so you don't have to) paints a fairly dismal picture. Around seventy-four percent of adults are overweight or have obesity—and the highest age group classified as obese is between the ages of forty and fifty-nine (forty-three percent). At no time are we more likely to gain weight than during the menopausal years.

"The most common complaint I hear amongst my midlife clients is that they've gained weight but aren't eating more," says Alyssa. "I feel as though I become the patient's detective. It's far more subtle than calories in versus calories out, as TikTok might have you believe."

Again, the aging process plays a part. Our body composition changes around this time (fat goes up, lean mass down). We need to accommo-date this and, to some degree, accept it. Retaining the body of a twenty-five-year-old simply isn't feasible (the stress!). From our thirties onwards, we lose between three to eight percent of our muscle per decade. Muscle burns calories with more efficiency than fat, so the more muscle you have, the higher your resting metabolism.

Then there's lifestyle. "A lot of us are moving less without realizing it," says Alyssa. "Think about it—as kids get older you don't run around after them so much. Perhaps as you've progressed through your career you have more time at your desk. Be honest with yourself." Mood can be another shift. When we're low, we might turn to food for comfort. As with alcohol, Alyssa suggests that if you're reaching for a packet of biscuits ask yourself whether you're hungry; she also emphasizes that we need to stop thinking about food as being a moral choice. "When we label food as 'bad' we then think of ourselves as bad and as having failed. Weight is incredibly com-plex and we live in a world where we try to simplify it." She also suggests that you might get your thyroid checked, as an underactive thyroid can also cause weight gain. Believe it or not, not *everything* can be blamed on peri- or menopause.

But they certainly don't help. At least fifty percent of us will put on weight during the transition. According to SWAN data, around two years before your last period, your rate of fat gain doubles and lean mass starts to decline, and this continues until two years after your last period. In doing the research around menopause I became more aware of such facts, changing my diet and cutting out the food I no longer process well. For the first time in my life, weight is not an issue and I've learned to love my small belly pouch, which is hopefully galvanizing news!

"Women's fat is stored around the hips when younger, and in perimeno-pause this storage moves to the belly," says Alyssa. Because fat produces estrogen, when levels go down our clever bodies store more fat around the middle to try and push it up. The British Menopause Society points out that as estrogen levels reduce, visceral fat (the fat around your organs, which you really don't want) increases from five to eight percent total body weight to ten to fifteen percent total body weight. Average weight gain dur-ing this time is approximately three pounds per year during the perimenopause transition, resulting in a total of around twenty-two pounds by the time menopause is reached. But hopefully armed with the right information you, too, can defeat the stats.

During perimenopause, it's thought that fluctuating levels of cortisol and estrogen may contribute to weight gain: stress hugely affects hormones, so reducing stress levels is important. Though the moment someone tells me something like that, I stress about how stressed I am.

"Lack of sleep is very common in peri- and menopause, because of night sweats, stress, anxiety, and insomnia, and this impacts the hunger hormone ghrelin," says Alyssa. "If you're short on sleep your body is trying to get its energy back. Because carbs are the number one fuel for the body, that's what you crave. We're triggered to want sweet ones because that's what the body recognizes as being fast energy." Take heart here—it's not your fault that you'd prefer to have a cake over an apple, but may I recommend making a few "powerballs" and keeping them in the fridge for those moments. Far better to stick a ball of sweet dates, dried fruits, and seeds into your mouth when the afternoon lull hits, and the hit lasts longer!

Body positivity is all very well up to a point, but excess body fat isn't a superficial consideration. It comes with a host of associated problems and risks, from heart disease, high blood pressure, diabetes, and certain cancers such as breast, colorectal, and kidney.

And yet dieting is one of the most depressing concepts ever, and a societal construct that keeps many women perma-distracted from relationships, career progression, or just having fun. Does anyone get to their last days and think, "I wish I'd stuck to the cabbage soup/apple cider vinegar diet and spent my life ten pounds lighter"? Hopefully not. Why do we have this perpetual desire to be smaller and to take up less space in the world? What's more, diets just don't work—out of the millions of Americans who resolve to lose weight every year, fewer than fifty percent will succeed.

Besides, sustained calorie restriction can lead to a slower metabolism, and nobody wants that! The best thing to do is take up permanent and sustainable changes to diet and lifestyle and ditch the self-loathing along the way. Aim to be strong, not skinny.

Bearing all this in mind, it's worth trying to eat the right foods. Alyssa recommends following what's called the MIND diet (Mediterranean-DASH intervention for neurodegenerative delay). This is a combination of the Mediterranean diet and the DASH diet (dietary approaches to stop hypertension), which has been shown to reduce the risk of Alzheimer's by more than fifty percent as well as hugely improving overall health. It sounds complicated, but really isn't (or I wouldn't suggest it). Basically, there's a focus on fruit and vegetables (including berries, nuts, and seeds), whole grains, lean protein, olive oil, and legumes, and you have a certain number of portions per week from each category. The recommended foods are packed with fiber, protein, and healthy fats. As I've said, I am incapable of following a strict regimen, but this list covers a lot of the things I love and isn't totally prescriptive. Red wine was on the original list of components but has since been removed. I'm afraid I'm old-school on that!

Intermittent Fasting

I wondered about the trend for intermittent fasting, which many of my friends are now doing with great (if smug) success. Here, you limit yourself to eating within a certain time frame—usually sixteen/eight (sixteen hours not eating and eight where you can eat) or eighteen/six. The idea is that when your body is fasting, fat stores are used as fuel. It's also said to support bone and heart health, metabolism and mental health, and there is some compelling evidence as to how it can improve insulin resistance.

"A lot of the scientific research has been done on men," says Alyssa. Forgive me for interjecting but . . . no surprises there! "Women are underserved, and the problem is that if you're eating within a brief six-hour window you might not be able to consume all the vital nutrients. Our body gets used to the regular mealtimes and primes our digestive system to start working close to those times, which equals easier digestion—something many women in midlife complain about." As someone for whom breakfast has always been more of a weekend treat and eating early only became a habit during the Covid pandemic, I seem to have become an intermittent faster by accident. Again, it does seem to have a positive impact on my keeping my weight pretty steady.

Protein Up

Most of us aren't eating enough protein, and the best diet tip I ever learned was to include it with every meal, especially breakfast. "It helps you feel full and it supports strength training and muscle building, which we all need to be doing at this time of life," says Alyssa. You need around 25 to 30g per meal, so one egg for breakfast (around 6g) isn't going to be enough, she says. "Protein recommendations will vary according to height, weight, activity level, and health goals. MIND emphasizes protein such as lean meats, poultry, fish, eggs, nuts, and seeds as well as four to five servings a week of legumes such as beans and lentils."

Sugar Tricks

Overconsumption of refined sugar is thought to be one of the drivers behind the current global weight crisis; on average Americans eat 60 pounds of sugar a year. Sugar is not the rocket fuel your body needs, nor is reducing your refined sugar intake rocket science. In fact, it's the bogeyman when it comes to burgeoning weight. "Glucose is the number one fuel for the body and brain, but it needs to be in slow-release forms so that we can function steadily (incidentally, up to twenty-five percent of our food is used by the brain)," says Alyssa. This means food such as oats, nuts, fruit, veg, legumes, and whole grains.

"There's always around a teaspoon of sugar in our blood, and our bodies control that. The food we consume is digested into simple sugars that fuel us. As sugar enters the bloodstream insulin allows it into the cells to be used as energy. But when there's a rush of sugar—a brownie (or two) for example—there's a corresponding rush of insulin to try and control levels in the blood. That surge of sugar goes down rapidly and leaves us half an hour later with low blood sugar and a desire to top up with another rapid release solution—a muffin or a doughnut." Back to those protein balls as a healthy and satisfying alternative.

Protein, fat, and fiber, including that in fruits, slow down sugar release so that blood sugar remains more stable. "If you're aiming to balance your blood sugar, eat protein before sugary or highly processed foods," advises Alyssa. Or I might add, avoid the latter two as much as you can!

Not only can sugar exacerbate menopause symptoms such as hot flashes, but there are links between hormones and insulin resistance, which might ultimately lead to type 2 diabetes.

Fruit and Fiber

If I haven't convinced you yet, read on. By increasing fruit and vegetable intake you might be directly alleviating your menopausal symptoms. In a large study from Australia, researchers found that menopausal women who ate diets high in vegetables and fruit (and the occasional glass of red wine) were twenty percent less likely to have hot flashes and night sweats versus menopausal women who ate high-sugar, high-fat diets.

Eating Your Estrogen

"The biggest dietary contributor to the relief of vasomotor symptoms is the inclusion of soy," says Alyssa. This contains phytoestrogens, compounds that can mimic estrogen. "If you aren't a soy eater, you might add it into your diet to see whether it makes any difference. You need to consume about a cup a day for at least three months—make your smoothie with soy milk and include edamame beans and tofu in recipes." Other foods containing high levels include legumes (lentils, beans, and peas). There's certainly nothing wrong with adding more soy to your diet regardless. Soy also contains protein, fiber, iron, and zinc, and a 2020 study pointed out that moderate intake of soy products is good for heart health.

Ultra-Processed Foods

Most importantly, keep an eye on what are known as ultra-processed foods (UPF), which tend to be lower in fiber and higher in unhealthy fat, sugar, or both. These are fast foods, fizzy drinks, sweets, burgers, sausages, many ready-made meals . . . you get the idea. They are rapidly processed by the body, meaning they can spike blood sugar. You also—and this is why calorie counting is a bit pointless—absorb more calories from UPFs than from simple foods. The body has to work harder to digest an apple or a Brazil nut. "I never say never," says Alyssa very sensibly. "Any food can fit into a diet if it's something you love. Even the MIND diet allows five servings of cookies or pastries a week. You just need to be aware of your consumption. It's the whole of your diet that matters, not what you choose to eat here and there." An absolute top tip, and I only recently stumbled on this, is to be active after a meal—even just five minutes of walking will benefit your blood sugar because muscles use the sugar up.

Your Microbiome

You might be wondering about the gut microbiome, which has also had a great deal of focus on it in recent years. There's certainly evidence to suggest that it changes during menopause. In November 2022, ZOE (a health science company) scientists in the UK published one of the largest studies to date to investigate gut bacteria during menopause. The study showed that postmenopausal women had increased levels of bacteria associated with inflammation and obesity. The conclusion was very much—as it so often is—that there's more research needed. Alyssa says that the best thing you can do for gut health is to consume a wide range of foods, especially fiber-rich and fermented foods—try adding live yogurt, kimchi, or sauerkraut to your daily diet. And she reminds us that "For fermented foods, it's important to purchase these items in the refrigerated section. If it's been made shelf-stable the bacteria is dead."

Weight-Loss Injections

And finally, to weight-loss injections or GLP-1 agonists like Ozempic, which affect appetite and metabolism. In theory, they are an excellent idea. Originally developed for those with diabetes, it was realized that they had an effect on weight. Demand has been so high that those who need the injections specifically for diabetes have struggled to obtain their prescriptions. In 2023, CNN reported that 1.7 percent of people in the US had been prescribed semaglutide for weight loss or diabetes (brand names Wegovy and Ozempic, though this doesn't have FDA approval for weight loss) that year, up forty-fold over the past five years.

"It's very nuanced. What I've learned from experts in the field is that they're a great tool for those who need to lose weight," says Alyssa. For those thinking of it as a quick fix, and I know you're out there, remember that these are still drugs, and therefore have potential side effects. It may seem unnecessary to point out, but without making cogent changes to the way you eat, these medications will only be a temporary fix. More data seems to be emerging about them on a near daily basis, including the suggestion that they need to be used long-term to maintain effects.

If you eat masses of high-nutrient, low-calorie foods, such as fruit and vegetables, this activates the same part of the brain as the weight-loss injections, turning off appetite hormones. Harder work, but a healthy and sustainable option! (As with anything, don't overdo it.)

The Wisdom of Supplements

I can't help feeling that menopausal women are a gift to the supplements industry, as we are often both vulnerable and desperate. I have seen some quite extraordinary concoctions advertised, especially on social media, and with very strange-sounding ingredients. These often purport to hold the secret to weight loss and amazing energy. Funnily enough—and I say this with deliberate sarcasm—if you ask to see their clinical studies, they rarely respond.

That said, I do swear by certain supplements, which I've carefully researched. I take daily vitamin D, B vitamins, a probiotic, omega-3, and a hair formulation that my friend the actor Gina Bellman recommended. This contains such hair helpers as zinc and selenium, and which I am sure has thickened my thinning locks.

Above all, I love magnesium. I generally have, within arm's reach, either magnesium spray, magnesium lotion, or magnesium bath flakes. It seems to help with sleep and muscle ache, but be careful to only take the recommended dose; I found that too much exacerbated symptoms, and my collection may appear to constitute product overload. But fellow sufferers of the debilitating condition known as "restless legs syndrome"—problems such as joint and muscle aches and pains are common in menopause—will know that there are few lengths to which we won't go to banish the symptoms of this little-understood condition.

My attacks start with a slight fizzing in my calves that swiftly becomes a brain-addling desperation to stretch my "restless" leg. When I was younger, it only struck when I was overtired or in cramped conditions. Plane journeys and nights at the theater were particular triggers. Now, there's no accounting for when the telltale signs will turn a relaxing night's sleep into a marathon of irritated wakefulness.

Rather than restful slumber, I'm leaping in and out of bed to try and stretch. Yet the minute I snuggle beneath the duvet, the symptoms return, often with a side order of agonizing cramp to make things even worse. A few years ago a friend recommended I try magnesium tablets and, within a few days of taking them, the worst of my symptoms had eased off. But still, there were nights when I was woken at two or three a.m., the telltale ache in my lower calves making sleep an impossibility.

That's when I added spray to my shopping list, and it's become something of a miracle cure for me. Magnesium can be absorbed via the skin, and a quick squirt on the affected area before I go to sleep means the worst of my symptoms are vanquished. On nights when there's time for a pre-bed relaxing bath, I pop in magnesium flakes as well. My other recently discovered miracle cure for those of you who are fellow "restless leg" sufferers is to wear compression socks when you feel a bout of this most infuriating condition coming on. I keep a pair handy in my bedside drawer along with my eye mask and silicone earplugs. The lengths a menopausal woman has to go to ensure a good night's sleep!

I asked Dr. Anna Barbieri, board-certified OB/GYN and integrative medicine physician, for her thoughts about the wild west that is the supplements landscape. She stresses that ideally we should get our nutrients via food, but the average US diet is deficient in many micronutrients and that's where supplementation may come in handy.

"Many women are very confused when it comes to supplements for menopause," she says. "On one hand, there is the constant marketing of lots of products with extraordinary claims but questionable ingredients, often backed by celebrities or celebrity doctors. Please do not believe the hype—often there is more hype to them than science." Here, I concur strongly, and would add that if something sounds too good to be true, it almost always is. "On the other hand," she says, "the message from the traditional medical system can be very broad and one-sided, too, and often rooted in a simple lack of knowledge on the part of a provider who tells a patient that 'no supplement' can work."

Dr. Barbieri's approach to supplements is, "Be skeptical and proceed with caution." If you are searching for supplements, they are, broadly speaking, divided into two groups. "There are 'hormonal' supplements such as phytoestrogens—plant compounds that chemically look a little like estrogen but are NOT," says Dr. Barbieri. "Unfortunately, the studies on them are often mixed and not of high quality. Black cohosh, for example, has not shown to make a difference in some of the better-designed trials, yet in others it does show efficacy." She points out that many women report improvement in symptoms when taking it, "So it may work for some individuals, and there's a wide safety margin."

The second group is "non-hormonal." "These are supplements that may reduce certain symptoms of menopause but do not exert their effect via a hormonal pathway. I often discuss this distinction, especially with my breast cancer patients as it is important for them in particular to avoid phytoestrogens," says Dr. Barbieri.

She reminds us that supplements including phytoestrogens are not comparable to MHT. "We cannot supplement ourselves out of menopause, which is why where possible MHT is the answer."

Any recommendations are likely to be based on where we are in the transition. In perimenopause, Dr. Barbieri says that too often we think of the obvious physical symptoms such as hot flashes and night sweats. "In early perimenopause, more frequent symptoms might manifest as irregular cycles, terrible PMS, disrupted sleep, and sore breasts.

"A potential supplement strategy in this group tends to look at the repletion of micronutrient deficiencies including vitamins and minerals—I usually check B12 and vitamin D in my patients." Many women need to increase their fiber intake, preferably via food, but if need be via supplements, she says. "Fiber is an essential nutrient for our microbiome—and science is starting to link a healthy microbiome to more optimal hormone levels.

"Supplements such as chasteberry (*Vitex*) have some evidence in the PMS arena, and evening primrose oil can be tried for breast tenderness. Ashwagandha, an adaptogenic herb, also has some data behind it for anxiety and sleep disruption." (These three are hormonal.)

As estrogen goes down, different supplements come into play. "Supplements with estrogenic activity include sage, which, although popular, doesn't have much evidence behind it, and it's the same with red clover and black cohosh."

"Soy isoflavones, particularly genistein and daidzein, are soy extracts that mimic the action of estrogen and have some evidence for alleviating symptoms such as hot flashes." (These can be bought in pharmacies.) There is also, she says, some evidence for the pro-estrogenic compounds pycnogenol—a French maritime bark extract—and rhapontic rhubarb, which is an extract from the root of Siberian rhubarb.

Then there are non-hormonal compounds. "Saffron can be effective in perimenopausal symptoms relating to mental health: anxiety, depression, and sleep as well as vasomotor symptoms. There's some evidence behind Swedish flower pollen for hot flashes—this is the main ingredient in a compound better known by its brand name Relizen. Finally, she says that inositol is a supplement that has some data regarding sleep and glucose metabolism.

You Might Also Consider . . .

. . . **collagen:** This is one of those supplements that is endorsed by many a smooth-skinned celebrity and does have some supporting evidence. "Many midlife women do not consume adequate protein and collagen in their diets," says Dr. Barbieri. "While I believe in dietary sources being of primary importance, there may be benefits to supplementing with collagen, especially if our food intake falls short of protein content goals."

She says that collagen supplementation is considered for two reasons: skin and bone health. "I frequently recommend it to my patients with osteopenia or osteoporosis for this reason, alongside lifestyle, vitamin D, calcium and exercise recommendations (as well as any prescription methods)."

Disappointingly, for those with or post breast cancer, she says that there's not very good data for either safety or risk. "We really do not know for sure if and how collagen supplements would affect risk of recurrence of breast cancer or therapy outcome." She recommends that women with breast cancer ("or anyone really") preferably gets their collagen out of healthy dietary sources such as bone broth or sardines.

. . . **vitamin D:** "The prevalence of vitamin D deficiency is quite high (up to twenty-two percent), and may be even greater in certain populations such as Black Americans and during winter," says Dr. Barbieri, who also reminds that we can only make vitamin D when the skin is exposed to the sun, and now we all use sunscreen—adding to the potential for deficiency. "Vitamin D has wide-ranging actions in the body. So I think routine vitamin D supplementation, especially in the winter, is something to consider. A dose of 2,000 IU of D3 daily is a safe level to take."

. . . **omega-3s** are considered essential fatty acids with numerous functions, says Dr. Barbieri. "They must be obtained through diet and supplementation." Best dietary sources are fatty fish, nuts, and seeds (for example flaxseeds and walnuts). "Unless you are the rare human with lots of omega-3s in their diet, and due to the wide safety margin on omega-3s— routine supplementation can be considered."

Top Supplement Tips

Dr. Barbieri says:

DO: Always check that whatever you take won't affect any medication you may be on, and if you are at high risk of breast cancer or are a breast cancer survivor then always ask your healthcare provider.

DO: Understand that supplements are not as regulated as medications, may have inconsistent or even harmful ingredients, and they may have side effects, sometimes serious, including liver injury.

DO: Look out for supplements with USP or GMP on the label—these connote greater quality. Also look for large companies that use third-party testing and invest in quality assurance and development.

DO: Try for three months to see whether they make a difference and stop after three to six (tops) months if there's none. (This doesn't apply to "maintenance" or prevention supplements such as calcium, magnesium, or omega-3s.) Women react differently to different supplements.

DO: Steer clear of proprietary blends that don't list ingredients or amounts—that's a big red flag. As are those with excessive claims about weight loss or "getting rid of all your symptoms."

DON'T: Overdo it. I often have patients who come in with a bag of twenty-five different bottles, where three or four could achieve the same thing or for whom a low dose of estrogen could be enough. Menopause management needs to be balanced, nuanced, and informed.

DO: Discuss supplements with your doctor and don't hide the fact you are taking them. I frequently "de-prescribe" supplements as an integrative medicine physician.

Thicken Your Bones and Muscle Up

This isn't an exercise book—as you will certainly have realized by now. But it's vital to mention physical strength. To my surprise, I've become a middle-aged cliché when it comes to keeping my body moving. I am dedicated to finding the time for a couple of yoga classes a week and Pilates, both of which I now do remotely on the miracle that is Zoom. I find that without having to make the trip to the gym I'm left with fewer excuses not to participate! I walk my dogs every day at a speed some of my friends find off-putting, and try to include a trot with a bunch of running mates once a week, though we go so slowly I have to admit it's more for the chat than the aerobic exercise!

Then again, mental health is also imperative and airing and sharing with like-minded companions can be a valuable route to keeping your spirits high. If I stop moving it has an immediate impact, my mood drops and my body stiffens up like an old twig. It's reassuring to hear experts say that no matter how sedentary a life you've led, and no matter at what age you start to move a little more, you will benefit from working out. Even increasing the amount you walk is good for you.

It's actually only in midlife that I've discovered that exercise is about far more than just getting your heart rate up. Exercise releases endorphins—the happy chemicals that push the mind into a short-term euphoric state. Not only does this alleviate low mood and help with anger, but it has a long-term impact on positive self-perception. In addition, it's a great way of counteracting loneliness. My running has become as much about spending time with friends (being sociable is definitely good for mental health) as it is about trying to fight the flab and my unstable fat/muscle ratio. What started as an effort has become an eagerly anticipated pleasure.

Like many women, having discovered how closely linked to our dwindling estrogen osteoporosis is, I'm haunted by the specter of weak bones, which is actually one of the biggest health concerns for postmenopausal women. At the age of fifty, I had a series of medical tests, including what's known as a DEXA scan to measure my bone density and when, as I've mentioned, I was found to be osteopenic.

"Menopause is the defining event in bone loss," says Dr. Andrea Singer, chief of Women's Primary Care, director of Bone Densitometry, and medical director of the Fracture Liaison Service at MedStar Georgetown University Hospital in Washington, D.C., and chief medical officer of the Bone Health and Osteoporosis Foundation. "Peak bone density is reached by the age of about thirty, and from that point the goal is to try and maintain it. In women, estrogen is protective for bone, and as it starts to decline so can our bone density." This loss increases through menopause—in the five to seven years after periods finally stop, women can lose up to twenty percent of total bone density, and we continue to lose it for the rest of our lives.

Osteoporosis occurs when the body has lost too much bone or can't make enough, or both, so that they are weaker and more likely to break.

"Around fifty percent of women over the age of fifty will have a fracture in their remaining lifetime because of it," says Dr. Singer. "It is a chronic disease, just like diabetes or hypertension, and requires lifelong management. Fractures can be life-altering events, and nobody wants to lose mobility."

There are many risk factors, and they will vary from person to person. Obviously, age is a factor—the older we are the more likely we are to have osteoporosis. "Having a fracture in adulthood and generally after the age of fifty increases the risk for future fracture, as does family history. Smoking, alcohol intake, and being sedentary are risk factors, as are certain conditions such as diabetes, rheumatoid arthritis, and medications such as steroids and aromatase inhibitors for breast cancer."

There are differences between ethnicities. The BHOF says that around twenty percent of Asian American and White women age fifty and over have osteoporosis, compared to ten percent of Latinas and five percent of Black women. "It's important, but it's only a piece of the puzzle," says Dr. Singer. "What's interesting is that although Black women have lower rates of fracture, compared to White or Asian counterparts, their outcomes following fracture aren't as good, and this can be due to lack of post-fracture screening and referrals for physical therapy and further treatment. It's not as simple as who has denser bones."

Although you'd think that early screening would be vital, it's not seen as such.

"The important screening tool is getting a bone density test, and a DEXA scan is the gold standard for diagnosing osteoporosis and osteopenia (the precursor to osteoporosis), which are also likely to be discovered when a fracture occurs," says Dr. Singer. However, some US guidelines (United States Preventive Services Task Force, USPSTF) say to only start having these at age sixty-five, and at a younger age only if there are one or more risk factors. A case of shutting the stable door after the horse has bolted, you might feel, as with so much to do with women's health.

"Many bone specialists, myself included, feel that if you wait until sixty-five you might have missed the boat, and that it makes sense to get a baseline around the time of menopause," says Dr. Singer. "There are many things we can do from a pharmacologic and medication point of view, but you can't treat what you don't know exists. There are some fairly well validated risk calculators to aid in risk assessment, but they are more robust when they include bone density. FRAX [fracture risk assessment tool] is probably the most commonly used; Garvan is another. It's far easier to treat and prevent further loss with early diagnosis." As ever, there is a shortsightedness to the approach. Far less expensive to do a DEXA scan than deal with a hip fracture.

The most important thing is to empower women to take charge of their own health, says Dr. Singer. "There are many things that we can do through our lifespan to support our bones, even as children and adolescents." Obviously smoking isn't good, and neither is excessive alcohol intake. We need enough vitamin D, and diet needs to contain building blocks such as calcium and adequate protein to keep muscles strong. "There's significant interaction between muscles and bones, and strong muscles also help to lower fall risk."

I am increasingly aware that muscle and bones go—if you will—hand in hand. Muscles support your skeleton, keeping you upright. Lose muscle mass and you become more likely to fall. Weight-bearing exercise is vital—not just aerobic—but also doing resistance work, with either bands or weights, because this helps stimulate bone remodeling and increased density. I keep suggesting that we do our running with ankle, wrist, or even weighted vests.

And the proof—if you will forgive the English expression—is in the pudding. Back in 2018, I visited Dr. Karen Hind, then assistant professor in the Department of Sport and Exercise Sciences at Durham University in England. She conducted an experiment with thirty menopausal women, none of whom were on MHT, to demonstrate the positive impact of exercise, especially weight-bearing, on your bones. I was pleased to discover that running, which I already enjoyed, was deemed one of the best forms of exercise for bone density. And, with a combination of MHT and exercise, I was able to reverse my diagnosis.

"We all need to pay attention to medications we might take or other medical problems that might contribute to bone loss or fracture risk," says Dr. Singer. "Estrogen is approved by the FDA for prevention of osteoporosis but not for treatment. However, we still use it in that setting—it clearly reduces risk of fracture by preserving bone density and preventing loss. For women who go through menopause early or prematurely, estrogen would be the drug of choice, and used at least until the age of natural menopause and perhaps beyond. There are other excellent osteoporosis medications that might be better for those who are very high risk or have already had a fracture; those that build bone, such as osteoanabolic agents, and those that work primarily to slow bone breakdown—called antiresorptive agents."

"I'm careful to look after my bones"

CANDICE, FIFTY-TWO, CEO, NEW YORK

I'm very careful to look after my bone health. My grandmother had osteoporosis later on, and my mother has had some falls, but not broken anything major. I have a background of thyroid problems and your thyroid can affect calcium levels, so I had bone density exams in my forties. Now I take a calcium supplement in the evening and have regular doses of milk, yogurt, and certain high-calcium vegetables such as broccoli. I also do yoga and Pilates and I have the most extraordinary OB/GYN who is eighty-seven. He talked to me about menopause, including how it can affect intimacy, and also offered MHT for bone health. I have used it for over a year.

"I drank too much wine"

KATE, FIFTY-SIX, CONSULTANT, VERMONT

I think that Mommy's wine time—something we all joke about—is a bit of a slippery slope for a lot of women, and I found myself turning to drinking more wine during my menopause. I know a lot of women of this age who've never previously struggled with alcohol, but now have a slight disorder.

My sleep was very disrupted from night sweats—I was uncomfortable from them and it took time to drop off again because my head would be full of things that were suddenly making me stressed. An unstable mind in the middle of the night is not ideal; it affects the whole day and impacts everything. I used to run a lot, but I didn't want to get up. I also had three teenagers and was working full-time. That combination led to low energy, some depression, and a change in my routines, which weren't helping my mental health. Now I'm trying to cut down on the wine and take back some control.

"I can't shift my excess weight"

CHRIS, FIFTY-FOUR, SPECIAL EDUCATION TEACHER, NEW YORK

For me the biggest symptom is weight gain, which started about four years ago. I'm not doing anything different but it's piling on, and I think I've gained about thirty pounds. I've always been a yo-yo dieter, but this is excessive, and no matter what I've done it just won't shift. I've pretty much starved myself and just started back at the gym. I'm unhappy and annoyed with myself, especially as I volunteer at an ambulance and am around lots of young people. The sensation of being ignored is hard, but I literally feel invisible. I've lost confidence in everything.

"Weight lifting has changed my body"

EMILY, FIFTY-TWO, NUTRITIONAL COUNSELOR, SAN FRANCISCO

I've really started to dedicate myself to exercise, and especially weight training, which I find far superior and impactful than doing cardio. I've always done a bit, but when the pandemic hit I couldn't work out at the gym, and did cardio at home. I felt that I lost muscle mass. Then the gym reopened and you could book in for an hour. I was like, I gotta go. I was really diligent about going five times a week, and as I spent more time there I started to lift heavier weights. It was a game changer. My body composition is far better than it used to be and my body fat is really low. It's good for my mood as well. I think more women should do it.

CHAPTER SEVEN

The Hell of Hormonal Insomnia

The other day, a friend whispered to me, "I think I've got that thing that you have." I was confused by the secrecy, mainly because we were alone in her kitchen. "You know, the thing . . . that sleeping thing." It turned out she was suffering from insomnia, but what she really meant was "I think I may be perimenopausal." Menopause and lack of sleep are as closely intertwined as a pair of young lovers. There, of course, any similarity very much ends.

I love my bed. Most evenings, I can't get there soon enough. I sink into a deep, virtually dream-free sleep, waking bright-eyed each morning, feeling healthy, energetic, and enthusiastic about the challenges of the day ahead. The night is my refuge and blissful darkness is where I retreat to regenerate and refresh.

Ha! If only. In reality, I love being horizontal in my cozy bed, especially with a good book, and I fall asleep reasonably swiftly. But by three a.m. I am usually wide awake. Most nights I know this because I've checked the clock three times since I first crept to the bathroom at one forty-five a.m. Within minutes of my return to bed, I feel the delicious fog of slumber evaporate, my heart rate rises, and my brain begins its relentless scanning for topics to fret about.

Occasionally, I am able to raise an exhausted smile from the banality of my "priority" worries. A thank-you note I failed to send a year ago, the bit part for a kitchen appliance I keep forgetting to order, how to take revenge on the annoying boss who patronized me by asking why I always wanted more . . . while seeking my advice on his own promotion, whether I booked a grocery delivery for Friday, whether it's still OK to love Alice Munro, the shirt my son needs, guilt because I didn't call my friend with breast cancer, where to go on summer holidays, how to get the car to the dealer for servicing, why the woman with whom I discussed documentary ideas hasn't replied yet, did I book a blow-dry slot on Tuesday, where's that blue dress gone . . . will the world end in my children's lifetime and should I give up wine?

I look again at the clock, it's three-fifteen a.m. and I'm getting closer to the moment when I'm going to either have to medicate or resign myself to staying awake. Instead, I add to my copious preoccupations: What do I have to do in the morning, and can I afford to be exhausted or should I resort to the cornucopia of drugs and sleep aids crammed into my bedside drawer for just this eventuality?

The only upside to this nightly game of insomnia roulette is that I am not alone, and I don't mean the company of a snoring bedmate, though I have that, too! The 2015 National Health Interview Survey showed that perimenopausal women were more likely to sleep less than seven hours in a twenty-four-hour period (fifty-six percent) than those who were pre- or postmenopausal, and it's generally reported that around sixty percent of women struggle with sleep around and after the transition.

Coincidence? I think not. This seems to confirm poor sleep as a symptom of menopause, less well recognized but just as ubiquitous as the hot flash. That said, it's a small comfort that there are thousands of us tossing and turning furiously. Misery doesn't love company that much.

We've included an entire chapter on sleep because I am obsessed with it. Not having had enough for nigh on two decades, whenever I'm fortunate enough to be dreaming, I dream about sleeping. Starting the day exhausted, anticipating only your return to bed, can take a stimulating timetable from challenging and fun to flat-out horrendous. Going to the office toilet and closing your eyes for a few seconds is pointless. There's nothing so thankless as trying simply to get through the hours of the day until you can fall back into slumber. I have been known to make my bed in the morning and whisper, "I'll see you later, my darling." Something I less frequently feel the compulsion to say to my husband or children.

In 2020, I wrote an article about what seemed to be an epidemic of sleeplessness, which appeared to affect women the most severely. Nothing I uncovered in the research process diminished my conviction that women in midlife struggle with one problem more than almost anything else: a lack of decent, restorative, regular sleep. To add insult to injury it happens during a period when restorative anything is high on the list of must-haves.

Insomnia was actually the first symptom of hormonal change that affected me, starting with baffling and frustrating nights of jerking awake and managing only fitful sleep afterward. During my years of poor sleeping, I've suffered from top-to-toe restlessness, from mind to legs. It's long been an expectation of later years that we sleep less. Just how debilitating and bad for us lack of sleep can be has only recently come to light. The most important thing isn't actually how brutal the next day can feel, but how vital proper rest is for our ongoing health. Not sleeping is linked to poor brain function, low mood, tiredness (obviously), and that other "s" word . . . stress.

More ominously, long-term lack of sleep has links to heart disease, type 2 diabetes, respiratory problems, dementia, and obesity. "It's vital for consolidating our memories, helping us learn new data, clearing out our brains and regulating appetite hormones," says board-certified sleep and integrative medicine doctor Valerie Cacho, who founded the website Sleephoria after seeing an increase in her practice of midlife women who were struggling. Our immune systems also need sleep. "There have been studies where people were given the common cold and those who were allowed fewer than six hours sleep had more symptoms manifest," says Dr. Cacho.

It's generally recognized that we need around eight hours a night, though there's no standard; between six and nine hours is enough for most adults. Those who sleep fewer than six hours a night on average have a thirteen percent higher mortality risk than those sleeping at least seven hours. So, not sleeping properly is actually risking my health and my life. It seems I dance a slow dance with Death every single night.

The Four Stages of Sleep

"I explain sleep by saying that it's where the brain waves slow down, rather like parking a car," says Dr. Cacho. "There are four stages of sleep: stages one to three are increasingly deep; stage three is deep sleep, or delta wave sleep; and the fourth stage is REM (rapid eye movement), when we have our most vivid dreams. We sleep in ninety-minute cycles throughout the night." As we age, we need less deep and REM sleep. Ideally, you wake at the end of a sleep cycle, when the body is naturally in a more awake state. "It's normal to have a brief arousal (*sadly not that kind!*) at the end of each cycle. Sometimes it's conscious and sometimes unconscious," says Dr. Cacho.

Sleep is regulated by two biological mechanisms. There's what's called Process C—our circadian rhythm, which is the twenty-four-hour cycle on which the body runs, and Process S, whereby what's called sleep pressure builds up in the brain during the day. "This is measured by the neurotransmitter adenosine, which increases as the day goes on," says Dr. Cacho. When you go to sleep, the pressure lightens." So the longer you're awake, the more adenosine you'll have, and the more likely that you'll be able to sleep. Incidentally, caffeine can block adenosine, which is why some people can't sleep if they drink caffeine late.

Turn Up the Heat: How Hormones Destroy Sleep

So, what's keeping us awake during our menopausal years? There are many factors at play, from pesky to-do lists to more tangible worries about children and parents, partners and careers, the burgeoning health conditions of midlife, and our fluctuating hormones. Estrogen, progesterone, and testosterone all play a part in the quality of our slumber.

"Hormones affect women's ability to sleep throughout their lives, from the point of puberty, through pregnancy, and finally menopause," says sleep expert Dr. Neil Stanley, author of *A Sleep Divorce*. He says there may be a simple explanation. "A recent paper suggested that the effect hormones have on sleep is merely because of the fluctuations in body temperature." Whatever the merits of his observation, only a man would say "merely" in that context!

"So your disturbed nights might be a consequence of temperature changes created by hormonal disruption," continues Dr. Stanley. "You need to lose around one degree of body temperature to sleep. Otherwise you're restless, uncomfortable, and fidgety. Women are hotter than men. It's as simple as that."

Your body perceives a rise in heat as being a threat. With your eyes closed, you don't know whether the house is on fire, or if you're hot because of hormones. Therefore, our natural defense mechanism wakes us up, and, for many of us, that's the end of it. Of course, in menopause, any temperature increase is likely to be thanks to night sweats. We are also likely to have lower levels of progesterone; this hormone can make you feel sleepy by increasing production of GABA, a neurotransmitter or brain chemical that makes you feel more relaxed and helps sleep.

The Sleep Foundation reminds us that insomnia is another factor; research suggests increased wakefulness means women notice hot flashes that they might previously have slept through. They also point out that our circadian rhythm is weakened postmenopause, meaning that sleep is affected.

A huge factor is sleep apnea (which concerned partners may call "snoring"). "As we age, the muscles in our upper airway naturally weaken," says Dr. Cacho. "In postmenopausal women hormonal changes impact the strength of our throat muscles." Obstructive sleep apnea (OSA), where the walls of the throat relax and narrow affecting breathing, is more common in postmenopausal women. It's been suggested that forty-seven to sixty-seven percent of postmenopausal women are affected. "As we age, OSA is associated with daytime sleepiness, headaches, high blood pressure, irregular heartbeat, stroke, and heart attack. Many people don't know they have it, but if you share a bed with someone, they might mention your noisy breathing or snoring."

Aching joints are also quite common throughout menopause. I found that, however tired I was, on some nights my restless cramping legs were able to counteract the exhaustion of my body, dancing an irritated little jig under the sheets.

Finally, the need to pee is keeping us up. Frequent urination in the small hours is called nocturia. The effects of estrogen are vital for the health of the urethra, bladder, and the pelvic-floor muscles. We discuss this in chapter ten, but needing to pee at night is more prevalent around this time—in one study, seventy-two percent of women aged forty-four to fifty-four needed to go at least once a night, and this can obviously affect sleep. So, if the flashes and anxiety don't get you, the poor muscle tone will! Another reason why using vaginal estrogen, still all too rarely prescribed or recommended, is absolutely imperative from perimenopause on.

I myself am no stranger to needing to pee in the middle of night or foolishly prolonging my wide-awake status by trying to "hold on" till morning. We all learn over time that the need to dash to the bathroom almost always overrides the possibility of dropping off again. Such is the wisdom that comes with age.

Some women are woken time and again at night. Once awake, overheated and drenched, you may need to change sheets or nightclothes, and, as sweat dries, you might feel cold. There are no positives. And then you might find you can't get back to sleep because of stress and anxiety, which might be related to hormonal changes, might be down to life stress, and might be a combination of the two.

The Stress Response

"Sleep is immensely complicated, and if sleep is disrupted you activate the stress response, which is fine in the short term, but long-term stress can lead to multiple problems," explains Dr. Russell Foster, professor of circadian neuroscience at Oxford University. He is also, incidentally, the man who discovered how our body clocks are regulated by light. My stress response is easily activated, I suspect, and it's not always to do with menopause.

"We may be the only species who can override the biological drive to sleep—but stress is the result," says Professor Foster. I have two dogs and can confirm that this is true. They can sleep absolutely anywhere and drop off simply by closing their eyes. I envy them this simplicity, although of course they don't have to worry about earning money to pay for the dog food. More confusingly, my husband, who does contribute to the dog food bill, appears to have the same ability.

When this stress response is activated, and for whatever reason, it all cascades in the wrong direction, like a game of Jenga collapsing. "Elevated levels of cortisol—the stress hormone—suppress the immune system, which predisposes to infection and, long term, even cancer," says Professor Foster. "Stress throws glucose into the circulation, leading to insulin resistance and a greater risk of type 2 diabetes. Sleep loss and stress lead to changes in the metabolic hormones ghrelin and leptin; ghrelin is the hunger hormone, and goes up when you're tired, and leptin, the satiation hormone, is reduced. The net effect is increased hunger, more calories consumed, and weight gain."

In summary, if you suffer from insomnia you may be fatter and more likely to get ill. Oh joy! "Many of us are chronically tired and desperate to sleep, but the biological drive for sleep is being overridden by the consequences of being stressed to buggery," he adds thoughtfully.

Not Just Estrogen

It's important to point out that the reasons for our midlife sleep deprivation aren't down to menopausal symptoms alone. There's a tendency to attribute everything to menopause, especially if your main source of information is the internet. ("Sore ear lobes, madam-of-a-certain-age? A graze on your elbow? That will be your hormones.") During midlife, or indeed any part of life, sleeplessness can be down to all sorts of factors. Menopausal symptoms are certainly one, but it seems relevant to include the other elements, because I find it reassuring to know, when I consider the continuing erratic quality of my sleep a good ten years after menopause.

"Sleep quality naturally deteriorates with the aging process," says Dr. Stanley. "Here, unusually, women benefit. Men start to lose the slow, deep-wave sleep, which is restorative, from around the age of thirty-five, and women from fifty-five. Obviously, when women have events such as menstruation, pregnancy, and menopause, it's hugely disruptive, but the underlying baseline doesn't shift."

This decline occurs because deep sleep has to do with memory, learning, and physical growth; vital for kids, and obviously less so for adults. We only produce human growth hormone (HGH) in this cycle.

"Men can't hunt or protect any more, because our knees are hurting," says Dr. Stanley. "We can still reproduce, but you don't need many men for that. Women are preserved by nature to both have babies and then to look after them." He says that this means women are more adaptive than men. "Historically, you had to deal with new threats to children and new alpha males in the tribe; that's why women can multitask—because they have to, and men don't." To be honest, he says, post-thirty-five, men are biologically redundant. You have no idea how cheerful it makes me feel to write this sentence! I pity them of course, but as a campaigner against women being made to feel redundant I can't help but welcome the fact that it's a slightly more level playing field. When it comes down to it, we humans might flatter ourselves as being complex creatures, but at baseline we are really nothing more than the need to reproduce and continue our species.

So it's possible that you can't go back to sleep because there's no physiological need. "It's not vitally important for the survival of the species." Men and women also have different circadian rhythms. For example, men are more likely to want to go to bed later than women—you may recognize this from the twenty-first-century phenomenon of Netflix watching. My husband is far more likely to say "just one more episode" than I am. This is also evolutionary, deriving from the time when women went to sleep with the babies and men stayed up later to ensure there was no danger. (These days, this state of defensive red alert is likely to be tempered by half a bottle of red and a couple of episodes of *Succession*.)

"From about the age of ten, men and women start to go to bed later," says Professor Foster. "Men peak at about twenty-one and women at nineteen and a half. Then they slowly move to an earlier and earlier time. But it's not until we're in our late fifties that men and women are getting up and going to bed at about the same time, and that's about two hours earlier than we did when we were in our late teens and early twenties. This is why asking a teenager to get up at seven a.m. is like asking a person in their late fifties to get up at five a.m."

When men do go to bed, they often disturb the lighter-sleeping women, who then struggle to go back to sleep. The general increase in obesity means men are more likely to snore or suffer from sleep apnea, especially as they get older, which is also disruptive. About forty percent of adult men are habitual snorers, though they are less likely to snore from the age of seventy onwards. There's something to look forward to!

So, while I diligently attempt to follow the advice I've been given and count my breaths to restore my equilibrium and compartmentalize the turmoil, my husband snores noisily beside me, deep in a contented sleep that not even the alarm clock can halt. If he knew how close to homicide this nightly inequity of rest brings me, he wouldn't be so relaxed. I counsel myself by remembering it's not his fault, but it's certainly not helpful that so many women's attempts to get back to sleep are challenged by their noisy partners.

"Also, on the plus side, sleep in women is designed to be relatively flexible from an evolutionary point of view," says Dr. Stanley. "They cope. So women are more able to recover from sleep deprivation, and also to rebound better from very little sleep. At the end of the day, men are there to protect and procreate; by nightfall, their job is done." I do love it when science confirms what you've always suspected! Lucky them.

Too Stressed to Stop

The other reasons for poor sleep at this time of life are, as you'd expect, because of our day-to-day stresses.

Not only are we busier than ever before, but the structure of the family has changed, and this has put more onus on women. "We've shifted from the extended family to the nuclear family within almost a generation and a half," says Professor Foster. "This means that childcare is no longer the responsibility of the extended family, but focused on the parents, and especially the mother. So the mother is on call all the time and this leads to awful guilt that you're not coping. We're not evolved to be able to cope by ourselves. In all primate societies, childcare is distributed across the extended family."

By the time you've reached menopause, this is quite likely to still be the problem. Small children are at least reasonably static, but the more they grow, the more they want to visit places. As the mother of two teenagers, I am not so much a maternal presence as an unpaid taxi-service-cum-laundry-woman and twenty-four-hour buffet provider, and I do this as well as working full-time. Ironically, despite these efforts, I constantly feel bad about not devoting enough time to them! A woman's work is truly never done.

This is also an age at which parents may need more support. I have many friends who are in the position of being at least a part-time carer—and that adds further stress no matter how generously you embrace that responsibility.

Our guilt or overwork translates to stress and therefore sleeplessness and, in some women, depression. "We know one of the destabilizing effects of sleep on physiology is that it increases the chances of being in a depressive state. Once sleep starts to slide, your physiology goes, your sleep gets worse, and the stress increases. The first sign of depression is a changed pattern of sleep," points out Professor Foster.

Think of all the distractions that surround us, as though we needed any other reason to stay awake. In the past, you put the last lump of coal on the fire and then went to bed. Now, we have 24/7 everything: TV, shopping, emails, social media, and work. Our evolutionary adaptation can't keep up with technology. Humans, and especially women, have more to distract us from sleep than ever. In fact, in 2017, then Netflix CEO Reed Hastings claimed that the streaming giant's biggest rival is our need for sleep. "You know, think about it, when you watch a show from Netflix and you get addicted to it, you stay up late at night," he said. It's designed for binge watching. That's why there are only a few seconds between episodes.

"Our individual sleep patterns are like shoe sizes," says Professor Foster. "One size does not fit all; some people need nine hours and others only need six. The key thing is to work out if you are a long or short sleeper and then try and defend your individual sleep needs."

We fret about waking up, but some of us don't automatically sleep through the night in one swoosh of eight hours. Instead, we might wake up once or a few times, and some of us may stay awake for a while.

Calling a Halt: The Solutions

The ridiculously long list of medications and supplements in my medicine cabinet proves that there's no simple solution. I take my daily MHT, which I believe helps—certainly if I forget to rub in my estrogel I pay a price in insomnia that night—and is another reason I have no intention of exploring the landscape of an MHT-free life. But as we've said, it's great, but it's not a cure-all. Some women find it resolves sleep issues but many others continue to struggle, with lifestyle factors and hormonal turbulence affecting us all uniquely.

I've also tried yoga breath counting (it often works, but some nights it proves impossible to stop the thoughts flooding in), CBD oil (quite helpful), having a bath with lavender oil (occasionally helpful), sleeping pills (very helpful, but I don't want to be addicted), white noise (better than just the sound of my thoughts rattling around), melatonin (in 2mg doses taken regularly, any more and I get nightmares) definitely helps, doing less work (aspirational but hard to pay the bills), and the Calm app (again, better than my own thoughts, but often they break through the ocean lapping soundtrack and scare me). Magnesium—oral or topical—is good for aching and restless legs, and I've found that my Kindle has been a godsend because it doesn't wake up my husband like switching on a light would, and after a few pages of reading my mind calms down and I generally nod off. "By the time women come and see me they have probably tried all the supplements and sleeping tablets," says Dr. Cacho. "They can certainly help, and we can always find a solution. But sometimes it takes a specialist to really delve deep." There is, she says, gender bias in sleep medicine. "Only too frequently, women are underdiagnosed, or misdiagnosed with conditions such as depression, thyroid issues, or insomnia, when the real issue might be OSA."

Just a few years of insomnia can feel like a life sentence and culminate in ruined careers, relationships, and quality of life, but thankfully there are solutions.

Treat Sleep

MHT

This has been shown to help reduce night sweats, which are the whispering fiery demons of the menopausal woman's night. Low estrogen is associated with less deep sleep, and progesterone helps you to relax and, as said, is known to increase the production of a brain chemical called GABA. Low testosterone can also affect sleep. "By the time women come and see me they've often tried MHT," says Dr. Cacho.

Lifestyle

Dr. Cacho says that certain foods can be sleep promoting. "High-fiber foods promote low-wave sleep, whereas processed foods and saturated fats cause more arousal and light sleep." And exercise during the day helps you to sleep at night.

Mind/Body Practices

"Mind and body practices such as mindfulness, breathing exercises, meditation, and gratitude journaling can all be beneficial," says Dr. Cacho. That racing mind that won't calm down is because our sympathetic nervous system is working overtime. "It's possible to learn how to strengthen this system and turn down the mind chatter in order to sleep." I've found that keeping a notepad by my bed to jot down the rare imperative chore or worthwhile inspiration I have in the early hours is also very helpful. Clinical hypnotherapy and acupuncture can also help alleviate hot flashes and improve sleep quality.

Sleep Clean

Apologies for adding this sleep hygiene advice, which seems terribly obvious. But it makes a huge difference to have a bedroom that meets your needs. Experts are quite correct when they recommend that your room be as cool as possible and that you wear natural fibers to wick away moisture, as well as using cotton sheets. "If you get hot and sweat stays on the skin, sweat evaporation is switched off, and you get hotter," points out Dr. Stanley.

Don't do anything before bed to increase body temperature: eating late, drinking too much alcohol, or doing vigorous exercise, although exercise during the day does help sleep quality. And we all know about leaving gadgets downstairs.

"Another—controversial—suggestion is not sleeping with your partner," says Dr. Stanley. "It means that you can have the duvet on or off, the window open or closed, and the freedom to toss and turn without worrying about disturbing them. This means you'll both get a better night's sleep and feel happier and healthier because of it. It might even strengthen your relationship." As with all things this is a question of compromise and balance, a good relationship being as conducive to restful nights as any medical intervention.

Very importantly, go to bed and get up at the same time every day. This maintains your body clock.

Bitter Pill? Melatonin

As day turns to night, the body produces melatonin, as one of many signals that it's time to go to bed. People with heart problems, on beta blockers, and the elderly have lower levels of melatonin, and this may contribute to the poorer sleep seen in these groups of individuals. Many of us take melatonin to aid sleep. A Sleep Foundation survey in 2022 found that 27.4 percent of people in the US take it. "Part of the problem is that sometimes melatonin works and sometimes it doesn't," says Professor Foster. "Some people seem to be quite sensitive to it and some aren't. All the evidence suggests that it isn't dangerous. The only thing I'd be careful about is if there is a family history of mental illness, as there is some evidence that it might lower mood."

Working It Out: CBT

"It's the frontline treatment for insomnia," Dr. Stanley says, and it's supported by the NHS, the EU, and the US. He says it's as good as, if not more effective than, sleeping tablets. "Whatever CBT process you choose, and you can pay potentially hundreds of dollars per session, remember that they all have the same components."

CBT (also see chapter five) is about reframing the fact that poor sleep is just a bad habit, and learning what affects sleep.

Naturally Tired: Supplements

There is some evidence of efficacy for valerian, passionflower, and hops. Passionflower is said to reduce brain activity and help sleep. Valerian has sedative effects, but nobody seems quite sure why—though it's thought it might be related to GABA production as well. And hops also appear to affect melatonin and the happy hormone serotonin.

"They've been mentioned since the fifteenth century, so purely on the basis of longevity there's certainly a belief that they work. Remember that, just because they're natural, it doesn't mean there aren't contraindications with prescription medication. Always check," says Dr. Stanley.

I know a few people who swear by Bach Rescue Night Remedy, which contains white chestnut, said to help switch off the mind from unwanted repetitive thoughts.

Dr. Cacho also recommends trying L-theanine, phytoestrogens, and chamomile. "This is interesting because some research shows it can be helpful for generalized anxiety."

There is some good evidence of magnesium's usefulness (see chapter six). It helps with leg cramps and muscle relaxation, and those who have trouble sleeping often have low levels of magnesium. Magnesium and melatonin together are said to be especially effective.

Obstructive Sleep Apnea

For those with OSA, sleeping on your side, weight loss, and what's called continuous positive airway (CPAP) therapy might all help, says Dr. Cacho. She also suggests that singing and playing wind instruments can help strengthen the muscles. "You can invest in FDA-approved home sleep studies to self-diagnose but the gold standard is laboratory diagnosis."

Sleep Trackers

"These are only so accurate," says Dr. Cacho. "A lot of people come and see me claiming to have insufficient sleep, but they've concluded that from their trackers." It is, she says, very hard to do sleep staging based on movement and heart rate variability. "Accuracy is somewhere between thirty and seventy percent. We like to use them for trends, but not for diagnostics."

Like so many aspects of our health, symptoms are subjective and the solutions we're offering aren't universal cure-alls. Hopefully, better understanding the contributing factors to any struggles you might be having with sleep will open the doors to finding the right answers for you. For too long we've simply shouldered the burden of our pesky biology and struggled on. Insomnia is a very real condition that can have a detrimental impact on all aspects of our lives, from relationships to mental and physical health, so it deserves to be taken seriously and tackled as a priority. Hopefully we've been able to offer you illumination on why you might be struggling and a toolbox to get you started on solving those issues.

"I'd fall asleep and wake at midnight"

JAMIE, FIFTY-FOUR, FUNDRAISING DIRECTOR, CHICAGO

In winter 2023, I noticed that falling asleep was fine but then I'd wake at midnight thinking irrational thoughts about trivial things: "Was I rude to someone? Is she mad at me?" I was very warm in bed, but that's happened all my life. It was affecting everything. I was tired, irritable, and very sensitive about things. My family noticed, especially my husband, who is a terrible sleeper. He'd wake up when I did. I went to see the doctor and she gave me Gabapentin, which has been really great. I'm feeling far less stressed about this stage of life.

"It was utterly debilitating"

MOIRA, SIXTY-FOUR, TEACHER, NEW JERSEY

The main menopause symptom for me, age forty-four, was being unable to sleep. I had severe hot flashes every night and every time I woke up it would take a little while to get back to sleep again. It was debilitating and I felt as though I'd gone through a personality change. I work as the head of a school, and normally I'm very patient, but I felt very tired, moody, and unable to concentrate. I didn't get any enjoyment from each day. After five months I went to my doctor and said that I needed hormones, which helped my sleep. I've now been on MHT for twenty years.

CHAPTER EIGHT

Women-Shaped Spaces

In October 2023, I found myself in a room packed with a handful of America's most successful businesswomen, gathered in a glamorous uptown venue amid the bright lights of New York City. It felt like a moment of tangible progress. Amid the clink of cutlery and the hum of chat, the atmosphere was best described as electric and anticipatory. At the front sat four pioneering campaigners for the power of midlife womanhood: Dr. Sharon Malone, esteemed OB/GYN, chief medical advisor at Alloy Women's Health, author of *Grown Woman Talk*, and friend of Michelle Obama. Naomi Watts, the Oscar-nominated actor and founder of brand Stripes Beauty. Pilar Guzmán, editorial director of Oprah Daily, and Joanne Stone, MD, MS, system chair of the Raquel and Jaime Gilinski Department of Obstetrics, Gynecology and Reproductive Science at the Icahn School of Medicine at Mount Sinai. A decade ago, such a stellar gathering celebrating menopause would have been an inconceivable event.

But since 2022, when I co-founded the campaign group Menopause Mandate in the UK, one of our key focuses has been pushing for change at work. Now, we were gathered to launch Menopause Mandate in the US, with Naomi as co-chair, and our Women in Work Summit (@WiWsummit)—a brand-new global forum bringing together industry leaders to talk about changing the toxic chatter, prevent the brain drain of brilliant women at the peak of their careers, and overall creating a female-shaped space in today's working world.

Pushing back against the man-made status quo began some time ago. It can't have been easy after the Second World War for men who came home from the battlefields to find women weren't just keeping the home fires burning but also gathering kindling, chopping down trees, running factories, and generally doing much of the "men's work" that had previously ensured their position as the "superior" half of the species.

We've all experienced the sinking feeling you get on returning somewhere familiar to find everything has changed. That's why I have some sympathy for those still clinging to the top rungs of the patriarchal ladder of success and trying to boot off the fifty percent of humanity who finally feel liberated enough to make their own ascent.

Not that women were exactly twiddling their fingers before then of course, but the economic model that's fueled the developed world since the Industrial Revolution is one in which success was predicated on the unpaid labor of one half of the population, making "going to work" possible for the other half. Even then, things might have returned to "normal" had the contribution of both sexes been treated with equal value. But, as has already been said, women's contribution to our evolution, from cave dwellers to conquerors and—small point—the survival of the entire species, has been downplayed since the dawn of time to make room for the elevation of those not strapped to the kitchen sink. It's important to bear this in mind when we look at the untenable situation in which we now find ourselves, where women have embraced the possibilities of fulfillment in realms aside from the domestic, and men are scratching their heads and wondering why we can't just seamlessly fit in.

So even now, the working world as we know it is entirely shaped around the male experience, unencumbered by periods and pregnancy, child-rearing, menopause, and all the other biological and fertility-related elements that make us ... well, female.

We've pushed, shoved, begged, demanded, and proved ourselves well beyond the confines of the domestic sphere, and proved time and again that we aren't just a welcome addition, but an absolute necessity to the economy, the evolution of society, and the future of our species and planet.

Yet our bodies are still perceived as something to hide, excuse, and compensate for, rather than accommodate and celebrate. Breastfeeding rooms and egg-freezing included in contracts are hard-won concessions, but all add to an omnipresent acceptance that somehow women are the problem, that we aren't quite the right fit, that we need to be molded and streamlined for the linear way work is conducted. *We* need to be accommodating—as ever.

For two decades, a slow-burn realization has been creeping up on me, from both watching and experiencing the ways in which women are penalized for their biology in their professional lives. It has become all too clear that it's not tweaking and concessions to accommodate our pesky differences that's required, but a full-scale revolution. Now we're in the twenty-first century, we need to have not just equality at work—which, by the way, we don't have—but equity. Once you add in women's indispensable contribution to financial progress, it's even more baffling that creating an environment in which all can blossom isn't a priority for all organizations, including the government. The inconvenient truth is that it's down to one irrefutable fact: we have different genitalia and accommodating ours means change must come.

Many of you reading this will be intimately familiar with the linear progression that defines success in the world of employment. A straight trajectory from school to promotion to retirement. But that route is the one created and enjoyed by men. Women, with our awkward biology, our different bodies, and the fact that we want "time off" for babies or fertility issues, simply can't squeeze our curves into that pair of trousers.

We do not fit a steady flight path, because that's not how two X chromosomes work, and that means that in the US almost one in five women has left or considered leaving a job because of menopause symptoms. It is nothing short of penalization for not having the "right" body parts!

In order to progress and embrace the challenges we face, a seismic shift is required in the way we consider women at work. Time's up on fine-tuning, instead we need a female-shaped space that fits us, not a small anteroom in which to discreetly conduct the messy business of being a woman. And nowhere is the division of the sexes at work more starkly in evidence than during menopause, a period of midlife when men are at the peak of their career trajectory and women are presumed to be plummeting off theirs.

Conversation around the subject of menopause in the office is—for the most part—swathed in shame, embarrassment, and full-on denial. Expert voice after article after report after study ad infinitum points out the urgent need for recalibration. In recent reports about menopause in the workplace, sixty percent of US women said they think menopause is generally stigmatized and eighty percent have cited symptoms as a workplace challenge.

Let's face it, if a cooling wind of change starts blowing through a woman's career during her late forties, it gets positively icy when she reaches her fifties. This might seem like a rather pleasant meteorological phenomenon for those of us who are feeling too hot half the time. But in reality the metaphor is less positive. Age, up to a certain point, is relative, but as you approach midlife it becomes depressingly defining, and the fact is that for most women the workplace might well become a more hostile environment as you head into your perimenopausal and menopausal years.

Frankly, it's a miracle that any of us have managed to break the glass ceiling. I sometimes feel as though I'm still tapping on it, like a bird outside a skylight, looking in on men roaring with laughter and bonding over profits and share prices. Effectively, women's life and health stages, from menstruation to menopause, are still woefully misunderstood in the office (or restaurant, hospital, or construction site). Our biology at work has been a very low bar for a very long time and has relied since time immemorial on that biblical misnomer that we are but a spare rib and a lesser version of men.

The glitzy dinner I described at the beginning of this chapter took place against the backdrop of Women in Work (WIW), the forum I co-founded in 2023, in response to the urgent need for a spotlight on women's health at work and in tandem their imperative economic contribution, backed up by ever-rising tides of data, all pointing out that we can't afford to sideline experienced women. Now established in both the UK and US, I'm happy to relay the message that companies can't afford to disregard the needs of female employees and that businesses benefit when women are included. Birthing WIW was both a dream come true and continuing evidence that there is a great deal still to be done.

Me and My Working Menopause

My own career history may be slightly unusual, in that I crawled back to my job within months of having both my babies. Much as I adored them, I struggled with the tedium of maternity leave after a full working life. Also, to be totally frank, as a freelancer with no prospect of maternity pay beyond the state's bare minimum, financial need also figured highly on my list.

Back in the earlier part of this century, I did once get told, via my agent, that a BBC TV boss felt that my "breastfeeding schedule" was not conducive to fulfilling my duties on *The Culture Show*, when I refused to commit to twelve-hour days. To my eternal shame, I did the "honorable" thing and stepped down. Aside from that encounter with a tragically unreconstructed hierarchy, while at the *Observer* and Radio 4, where I worked for twenty years with an almost entirely female team, I always felt I was one of a gang trying to navigate the same terrain.

Further up the bureaucratic chain, I would be lying if I said the same were true. As I headed toward fifty, attitudes started to change. Even with my skill set unquestionably improving with maturity, I stopped being considered for any of the coveted presenting positions that came up. It was increasingly obvious that those in a position to promote me were wondering instead when I might gracefully accept retirement and remove myself as an obstacle to their pursuit of a younger listenership. Your fifties, it became clear, no matter how you dressed it up, were just not the right age for advancement, and especially not if you were a woman.

When I wrote in exasperation to my then boss, his response was to ask in frustration why I wasn't simply grateful for my thirty-minute, three-weeks-in-every month, book show. The idea that I might have larger ambitions or want to work on a more full-time and challenging basis was clearly absurd. The expectation of gratitude for a job you have actually earned is yet another inequality between the sexes! What's more, like all women, I somehow blamed myself, rather than pointing my finger at a misogynistic workplace culture.

It is hard enough being an older working woman in an ageist society with a youth obsession. But if menopause is simultaneously robbing you of your confidence and sapping your energy for the battle, it's even harder to stop yourself being crushed by the tsunami of society's expectations. As increasing anxiety and sleeplessness took their toll in the couple of years from forty-nine to fifty-one, I found plenty of indignities and fears to flood my late-night subconscious and keep me from slumber.

At work, in a blur of sleep deprivation and assailed by mysterious symptoms of stress unrelated to the actual pressure I was under, there were moments when I was desperate to take a sick day. But what was my ailment? And had I known it was menopause-related, would I have dared to highlight my condition? I've already discussed the less-than-supportive attitudes I encountered when I became a mother. Did I really want to throw myself on the mercy of similar patriarchal platitudes? Back then, I wasn't sure any woman had ever claimed a day off for menopause (I'm sure it happens, but like debilitating periods, under cover of "food poisoning" or something similar). For so many of us, the path of least resistance is the least confrontational choice, so we accept our fate, fade to gray, and disappear from view.

Until recently a key reaction to a woman who has the temerity to be openly suffering from menopausal symptoms was either sniggering or an awkward silence. That's why so many of us are still paralyzed at the prospect of public humiliation, when hot flashes might turn us briefly into the crimson, sweating victims of hormonal imbalance. The thought of periods is still enough to make many flinch, but at least they mean you are ripe and fecund. Periods stopping because of age (yuck), along with being hot, sweaty, dry, agitated, exhausted, and embarrassed . . . Well, it hardly bears thinking about.

It was over a decade ago when my symptoms started, and happily there have been some improvements to the discourse and the conditions. Back then, there was scant possibility of citing brain fog as a valid reason for taking a moment. To my surprise, our evolving attitudes to menopause at work might be one way in which the UK could be called "world beating."

This is not to say that our offices are a mecca of understanding, with open windows, quiet zones for a five-minute meditation, CBT instruction in controlling hot flashes, free fans on every corner, and flexible hours for all. And there are still many examples of gross unfairness. But there is also brilliant campaigning, legislation, political engagement, and a growing acceptance among all ages and sexes that menopause is an inevitable experience and that, as invaluable members of the workforce, women might need a bit of support.

So, armed with the experience of successful and ongoing campaigning in the UK, we decided to export what we've learned and delve deeper into the situation stateside. How are menopausal women treated in the workplace here, what are the changes that are taking place, and what further improvements do we still need to demand in a world that remains surprisingly resistant to creating better conditions for our curving career path? Back to that female-shaped professional space for working women. And, from a prosaic point of view, is doing so—let's be blunt—going to improve your career opportunities and make you more money or as doubters fear, speed you to redundancy, and worse?! Perhaps even more importantly, what's in it for business because doing the right thing, if it has an economic imperative, is always that bit more compelling in a capitalist world.

The Cool Crowd: Menopausal Women at Work

First of all, here's a dismal overview of the facts. These highlight just how resistant the working world remains to women's entirely reasonable requirements.

The US Bureau of Labor Statistics reports that 41 million women over the age of forty are currently working. This means that menopausal women represent twenty-six percent of the workforce or, to put it bluntly, one in two working women is menopausal and therefore, whether you like it or not, we're vital cogs in every wheel of the economy. Imagine what would happen if we went on strike! Everything would collapse. I was mighty jealous when Icelandic women actually did it in 2023 to push for the pay gap to be closed and for action against gender-based violence, this having been my dream global "celebration" for International Women's Day for years.

But back to reality.

A 2023 Mayo Clinic study of 4,440 women (Impact of Menopause Symptoms on Women in the Workplace) found that thirteen percent of women reported at least one adverse work outcome as a result of menopause symptoms—such as missed days, reduced hours, or even being fired.

Much of this is due to a general lack of education around menopause, but also because there isn't support from employers. "Break Through the Stigma—Menopause in the Workplace" is a 2023 report by the Bank of

America. It reveals that although seventy-one percent of employers have a positive perception of their company's culture toward menopause, only thirty-two percent of women employees share that perspective.

Now, reports and studies and surveys are all very well, and because they look at different demographics, age ranges (within the menopausal spectrum), and sizes of groups, it's hard to take single statistics as absolutes. But in the last few years there has been an ever-growing pileup of such studies, all broadly reporting the same conclusion: that midlife women are suffering at work, that many are leaving, and that it is costing companies dearly.

On this issue, today's data-driven focus is truly our friend. Menopause symptoms are costing an estimated $1.8 billion in lost working time per year according to the 2023 Mayo Clinic study, a staggering statistic that has been globally quoted since its release.

"I anticipated that we would see a relationship between adverse work outcomes and menopause symptoms based on what we hear from our patients in clinic," says Dr. Juliana (Jewel) Kling, chair, Women's Health Internal Medicine at the Mayo Clinic in Arizona, who was part of the study team. A woman after my own heart, she continues, "It's important to show in numbers what we're already seeing to be able to highlight opportunities and effect change."

As with anything to do with women's health, there are further inequalities when it comes to race and wealth. In that same Mayo Clinic study, it was reported that women of color are disproportionately affected, with Black and Hispanic women more likely to report an adverse work outcome related to symptoms than their White counterparts.

In the UK, although we are seeing progress in many organizations, if you're working part-time or freelance, you are arguably far less likely to be in a company with any sort of menopause policy, or even acknowledgment of the subject, and little hope of financial support should you be unwell. It's not too much of a stretch to suggest that it's the same in the States, where menopause policies are still a relatively new concept. In a recent survey, just fifteen percent of large organizations said they offer or plan to offer specialized menopause benefits (though this is up from only four percent the previous year).

What's more, although 4,440 women were surveyed in the Mayo Clinic paper, Dr. Kling points out that these were women with access to the Mayo Clinic or who were receiving primary care. "So the results aren't entirely representative of marginalized women or women that might not have access to care, which probably means that those numbers are vastly underestimating the impact."

She adds: "I work in a clinic where we see women who don't have health insurance, and oftentimes there is no option for them not to work; they're either the breadwinner of the household or they're running the household and just have to push through, and don't have resources. And if you have no access to healthcare services or treatments, this will negatively impact on future health and longevity.

"It's a double-edged sword, because we don't want menopause to be demonized and like a disease that women need more time off for. All women go through menopause and most have symptoms. It's about creating space to discuss and acknowledge and then empowering women and their clinicians with tools that are effective to help."

Benefits to Companies

I mentioned the appeal of the profit margin. A rather magnificent piece of research called "Woman Count 2020" was conducted by the Pipeline, a gender-diversity consultancy. They found that FTSE 350 share index companies that had at least thirty-three percent female membership on their executive committees had a net profit margin of 15.2 percent, while those with no women had a net profit of just 1.5 percent. That means that firms with no women on their executive committees missed out on $60 billion in a year.

According to the 2015 McKinsey Global Institute Report, $12 trillion could have been added to Global GDP by 2025 by advancing women's equality worldwide—at today's tortoise-like rates it will take 151 years to close current gender gaps. Unbelievably, despite the evidence for it being a sound investment, only two percent of venture capital funding goes to women.

That 2023 "Break Through the Stigma: Menopause in the Workplace" report also showed that women with access to menopause benefits felt they had a positive impact on work, and eighty-three percent of those working in companies with menopause benefits would recommend their company as a great place to work, compared to sixty-nine percent with no menopause benefits. When women leave the workplace, as they are doing in their hot and sweaty swathes, it's costing thousands to replace them. So, more women = more money. In the words of that oft-quoted, but genius, hair advertisement: We're worth it.

Sitting Pretty: Sexism at Work

It's hard to miss gender inequality. Let's face it, as you head toward the top of the tree, smashing glass ceilings and blue-skying your ass into the boardroom, you'll more often than not find yourself awash in testosterone.

Sadly, of course, not everybody in charge of a company is prepared to employ people on merit rather than on the basis of having a penis rather than a vagina. That's all sexism in the workplace comes down to, unless the suit in question is also employed on the basis of what friends you have and which esteemed school you attended. Here, I know that men also feel the injustice of the assumption that wealth and education equals brains and the ability to lead, which I think we all know is very much untrue.

I say all of this as someone famed and employed for my own voice, but my husky tones were honed in a series of Irish state schools rather than any Ivy League educational establishment.

"What most companies don't understand is that one-fourth of the workforce is either in perimenopause or menopause and their symptoms aren't being addressed," says Dr. Mache Seibel. "This is not only bad for female workers, but it also affects employee retention and satisfaction and the company's bottom line." He calls menopause at work the "silent ceiling," a metaphor I think very apt, and brings to mind women in danger of concussion from bashing against an invisible barrier.

"We have a situation where there isn't an appreciation that the businesses are contributing to the loss," he says. "Breastfeeding has now become something that businesses understand is important, but the understanding of menopause is a bit of a mystery. It's complicated by those who are misinformed, those who are uninformed, and those who are informed but are afraid they'll say something wrong. So there's just discomfort or ignorance or not caring enough."

Dr. Seibel was involved in a 2023 survey that examined the impact of menopause in the workplace. Seventy-nine percent of women were experiencing problems with sleep; seventy-eight percent were struggling with brain fog, concentration, and memory; and sixty-six percent suffered fluctuations in mood.

"These symptoms do not create the ideal résumé for someone who has a highly impactful position trying to organize others," he says. "If businesses could conceptualize that helping women would save them from losing staff, that there would be increased performance, job happiness, satisfaction with their work, and self-confidence in terms of being mentors for younger women . . . perhaps they would be more open to supporting midlife women. But, at present, they overwhelmingly don't."

As my kids say, charmlessly, and without looking up from their phones, you do the math. It seems quite evident that, from an employer and employee perspective alike, menopause needs to be acknowledged and respected in the workplace. Like food for hungry children, it shouldn't have to be argued. If you're a business, it makes financial sense to look after your employees, no matter what hormones govern their health.

Work and the Law

I am positively haunted by the following tale. In 2017, a 911 operator named Alisha Coleman won a settlement against her employer after she was fired when—and it's worth using official wording here, "she accidentally soiled company property due to heavy premenopausal menstruation." In other words, she experienced bleeding that soaked through her clothes onto a chair. Rather than expressing the only obvious reaction—enormous sympathy—the company first disciplined her and then, when she subsequently and accidentally (obviously) bled onto a carpet, they fired her, even though she had cleaned the carpet. The reason? Again, let's use the stark official wording: "She was terminated for failing to maintain high standards of personal hygiene." That this could happen in a civilized country beggars belief.

"Women are covered by the Pregnant Workers Fairness Act," says Marcy L. Karin, the Jack & Lovell Olender Professor of Law and director of the Legislation/Civil Rights Clinic at the University of the District of Columbia. Professor Karin says that this means workers can ask for what are known as reasonable accommodations. "I'm a lawyer and a law professor, and I can read the text. The Act offers reasonable accommodations on the basis of pregnancy, childbirth, or related medical conditions. Well, perimenopause and menopause are related medical conditions.

"It means that workers might be able to request a uniform modification. They might ask for access to a wellness room, or to take a break or have an additional break in order to use restroom facilities more often and without getting fired or disciplined." It seems so simple, but, she says, there are countless stories in the US where people have been denied bathroom breaks or other simple adjustments. The only problem, apart from the Act not mentioning menopause, is that it seems unlikely that women will necessarily know that this Act exists and applies to them.

Returning to Alisha Coleman, her story did end happily, and personally I hope that she is living out her life in a five-star location in the sun. But when it comes to protection at work, the situation is perhaps best described as "vague" should you wish to challenge your employer. There are a few tribunals, but these are few and far between. This is for a number of reasons.

"Alisha was comfortable talking about what was happening and was willing to keep fighting," says Professor Karin. "Generally, menopause isn't a complaint that people raise, because they assume there's no protection." This means, she says, that women might have to carry a used tampon through a store because there's no bin in the toilet. "Or they're out on a rig and there's no access to a women's bathroom or water to wash their hands after using a menstrual product." Women deal with it, she says. Imagine the humiliation of having to explain or ask: "You're going to use makeshift menstrual products, or use antibacterial hand gel." There is, she says, a growing realization that it's not OK to have hot flashes dismissed just because their boss's wife didn't have any.

So, *would* you take action at work? Probably not. Menopause falls under a number of different laws that provide protection against harassment, bullying, and discrimination on the basis of age and gender, but it's rarely specifically mentioned. "On the federal level alone, it's under the Age Discrimination in Employment Act," says Professor Karin. "It's Title VII of the Civil Rights Act. It's the Americans with Disabilities Act. It is also about rights under the Occupational Safety and Health Act and the Family and Medical Leave Act. And there's state equivalents that might offer different protections, as well as the right to reasonable accommodations under the Americans with Disabilities Act and the Pregnant Workers Fairness Act.

"You effectively have something that nobody, or very few people are talking about, something that is causing you to have to choose between your physical and psychological health and your economic security, and that you feel it's worth rising to the level of asking or pushing back or insisting that your rights be enforced." There is, she says, some union activity. "But you're going to feel as though you're by yourself, and talking about things that nobody else is talking about to people who don't have the same lived experience. And you're going to need to be able to afford to fight. At the end of all this, the remedy you're going to receive is not going to be in proportion with the time and energy expended." Still feeling ready to take on the role of Erin Brockovich, the Menopause Years? Thought not.

Who Is Helping?

Interestingly, the lack of support appears to be partially down to a lack of communication. The Bank of America report also reveals what they call a "number of disconnects" between how employers think they're supporting workers, and how workers feel (oh to be a fly on the wall in those conversations!). More than half of women do not feel comfortable discussing menopause in the workplace because it feels too personal, which appears to have led to only fourteen percent of employees saying their employers recognize the need for menopause-specific benefits, and the primary reason employers don't offer menopausal benefits is that employees haven't asked for them. It's a brilliant report, but there's an awful lot of stating the obvious, which, clearly, if depressingly, needs to be spelled out.

Perhaps this isn't surprising. As we know, many of the trickiest symptoms are also the most subtle, such as anxiety and brain fog. If these occur in the office—forgetting things or worrying about completing deadlines—

it's hard to know whether it's just life stress and general pressure or a pesky period of hormonal change. Or both.

Hot flashes make it easier to identify what's happening. But a surge of red-hot heat rippling through your body as soon as you are stressed means that having a meeting or making a presentation in a room full of colleagues is pretty daunting. The all-consuming fear is that you'll wind up highlighting the very thing you're trying to disguise. Further mentioning it as being a "problem" in a one-to-one with a line manager is near inconceivable.

I am writing this book aged sixty-one. Having worked since the age of sixteen, I have been perimenopausal or postmenopausal for around a quarter of my working life. Yet despite some pretty desperate days, following nights of palpitations and insomnia, and the low mood that often comes with lack of sleep, I've never once had a day off to facilitate my menopause. That's not a boast, it's a lament for me and the millions of women out there who struggle through debilitating symptoms, while juggling their domestic and career responsibilities and trying to look as youthful as possible so nobody notices they're middle-aged.

Are Women Weak?

In early 2024, there was a post doing the rounds on LinkedIn quoting a headhunter saying that he'd been asked not to put forward any applicants over the age of fifty, as potential employers assumed that such qualities as energy, talent, and hunger for new horizons were unavailable in the skill set of this age group. It very much exemplifies many attitudes only too often held about midlife women at work.

As I've already said, on every measure the data available contradicts that outdated notion. I firmly believe that we are more ambitious; equating maturity with tired and unenthusiastic is simply bad business. The extra stresses placed on us at this time, such as kids and elderly parents, may mean we are under pressure, but not that we are less driven or indeed less able to do our work. We are the only people suffering. Menopause has been called "the third shift" by some, as we juggle office, home, and hormones.

But isn't there—and you may have been thinking this for a while now—a bit of an argument emerging for simply not employing menopausal women? This attitude is a concern that has been voiced time and again by women to whom we've spoken. It's bad enough getting older in a youth-obsessed society, never mind going through a transition that positively marks you out as having one foot in the grave.

In the UK, employment protection for menopausal workers is covered by several acts, including the Health and Safety at Work Act (1974) and the Equality Act (2010), which could cover menopausal women because of gender, age, and disability. Women who go to the courts in the UK when they are treated unfairly because of menopause have to shoehorn their claims into one of those categories. Not only do women need to keep their bodily functions under control in the workplace, but we also have the burden of finding an appropriate category for making a tribunal claim!

And this means that women may actively object to workplace menopause conversation and education, because asking for time off, fans, and access to toilets and showers makes us look unemployable. Many feel that you might as well start a conversation with the words "Let's talk about why I'm no good to you. Hire a man instead."

There has even been a study showing that workers perceive women described as being menopausal as less confident and emotionally unstable. (However, another study revealed that honesty about menopausal status meant women were seen as more leader-like.)

Few of us would be comfortable sharing with a senior male colleague that they might need someone else to do the presentation to the new clients, for fear of fueling the idea that women aren't able to do a job as well as men. The debilitating symptoms might be taking their toll, but does it sound credible, let alone professional, to be excusing yourself from work because your hormones are in turmoil? This is with the caveat that on a good day you'll probably be twice as good at that presentation than you would have been in your thirties! Good women are being lost because they are having bad days, which makes no sense on any level.

Putting the "Men" in Menopause

Allyship from men in the workplace is also vital. "Of course men should be part of the conversation about menopause," says Keith Lieberthal, a management committee member at an elite advisory firm in New York City. "I think we've come a long way in beginning to understand from a childcare and birth perspective, but I don't think the conversation's advanced yet when it comes to the reproductive cycle, and men need to be a part of that."

Current statistics estimate that men head up over sixty percent of American businesses. "So whoever runs the company has to be responsible. Of course, in a knowledge business like ours, talent is your most important asset and decisions that enable you to retain the best of half your talent pool over the course of their careers just make good business sense. But the cultural message is also important. Particularly at the high end of the talent pool, people are looking for places that reflect values beyond just the commercial mission of the organization. They want to look at a firm and say: 'This place cares about its people, not just its profit.'"

Data Drive

The word "FemTech" was coined by Ida Tin, a Danish entrepreneur, back in 2016 and it is playing a significant role in tech and innovation that provide solutions to women's health problems. Tin saw an opportunity to help women take control of their health, and founded Clue, now one of the most popular period-tracking apps in the world. Apparently the word "FemTech" is used to reassure investors (and prevent male embarrassment!?). Rather than saying "we've invested in a menopause app" they can say "we're invested in FemTech." I'm not sure what the gender equivalent of greenwashing is, but . . . ?

Anyway, FemTech is very welcome. There's Alloy Women's Health, which offers online menopause advice, care, and medicine. Maven Clinic was the first female-focused tech start-up to be valued at over $1 billion; MiDOViA supports employers and employees to understand menopause and create long-lasting and sustainable change—CEO and co-founder April Haberman says that both men and women attend their workplace seminars; and Peppy Digital Health App provides workplace menopause support. A 2022 McKinsey article says that FemTech is filling in some of the gaps. "Deploying technological and consumer-centric solutions to address menopause can serve as a model and an enabler for future female leaders."

Working Toward the Future

I believe numbers and data will finally change the way in which the working world is structured for women. Half the population wishing for their biological needs to be accommodated is obviously an unreasonable ask (I speak with heavy sarcasm). But cold hard financial facts about economic success surely cannot be denied, and at the moment they're stacking up like a game of Jenga to provide irrefutable proof that in order for your business to thrive, you need to consider your female employees.

There needs to be structured and universal support in all organizations as a matter of course. "There's so much that needs to be done," says Dr. Kling. "It's probably best addressed from multiple fronts. The first important step is that we're talking about menopause, and creating a space for women to recognize that what they're experiencing is also being experienced by many other women, and that it's OK to talk about it or to seek care."

It's encouraging that progress is happening, although it's currently creeping along rather than taking off and soaring into the skies. As fifty percent of the population is going to go through the menopausal transition, I refuse to feel any gratitude for any "concessions," as I firmly believe them to be a human right. *Of course* we need to ensure that women are comfortable at work.

There are many companies paying lip service to the concept of menopause-friendly workplaces. And it's a start. But, returning to my original point, "menopause friendly" isn't good enough. It's not acknowledging the real problem, which is that the workplace isn't designed for the female of the species, and that it needs to change on a large scale and in a permanent fashion. The value of mature, professional, and committed women in the workforce, eager to throw themselves into new challenges, needs to be recognized, celebrated, and embraced, and the workplace resized to fit us all.

"The need for change"

ALEX MAHON, FIFTIES, CHIEF EXECUTIVE OF CHANNEL 4, LONDON

I had not realized how impactful and dreadful menopause was in women's lives until my eyes were opened to it by a couple of women I know in their fifties and sixties. And then I realized that utterly brilliant and experienced, and thus very valuable, women were leaving the workplace because of a health problem—albeit a temporary and fixable health problem, and one we will all experience. And that the onset of the health issue was coinciding with caring pressures, sometimes happening far earlier than expected, and often coinciding with a real and common life stage where one wonders if one is still attractive. This stage is hard for men, too, and is notoriously often tackled for them with a Porsche/golf trip/second wife. But it isn't even talked about for women because of embarrassment and shame, and a somewhat pathetic lack of ability to address issues to do with women's health in our conversations.

And then this seemed a pointless, unfair, and discriminatory perspective, and one I noted was a real taboo in the workplace. An utter taboo. A pointless taboo. And I thought that that kind of discrimination isn't right.

I realized we could make a big deal about it and get big coverage (I didn't clock quite how big!) if I announced it all as a female CEO, and I realized that, in doing so, lots of people would make assumptions about my age, or ask me if I was in early menopause, if this was personal, but that taboo was in and of itself worth tackling.

"Menopause at work is shunned"

HEIDI DIAMOND, SIXTIES, ENTREPRENEUR, NEW YORK

There are companies supporting fertility, but menopause is still an out-there concept with the general population. (Until you get groups of women together, that is!)

I've been an executive for many companies, but can't think of any occasion where someone came to me in distress because of perimenopause or menopause, or any time when a woman said that they were desperate or "I'm in bed. I feel like I'm on fire and I'm heading for an ice-cold bath." I have had women saying they need a mental health day, and the underlying issues were clearly menopausal. I think it's mostly because women just grin and bear it, although Millennials and Gen Z seem to be outspoken about everything. But my generation, and the women coming up behind me . . . if you had a cold, you worked. If you were sick, you worked. You stayed home only if you were really ill.

I have a colleague who went through breast cancer treatment and never missed one day, even through chemo and radiotherapy. There's a lot of genuine suffering in silence.

"It's tough to be a woman aging in the film industry."

KAM HESKIN MABY, FIFTY, FORMER ACTOR, LOS ANGELES

I had both my kids in my forties and feel as though that may have possibly reset my hormones. I met my husband at age thirty-nine, and had my first son after IVF at the age of forty-four, then my second son I had naturally at age forty-seven. Before they came along, I was starting to have hot flashes, but now my periods have returned. I feel like a bit of a unicorn! It's nice to feel younger—it's not easy getting older in LA, and Hollywood is a tough industry to age in. I certainly noticed that I was getting different parts once I hit my late thirties and early forties. I decided to take a step back and forge a different path. I feel very blessed to have my family.

"I almost lost my job"

ERIN, FIFTY-FIVE, PUBLICIST, NEW YORK

I've had depression most of my life, and around fifty-one, when menopause kicked in, I started to become manic, where I'd stay up all night doing pointless research on the internet about random bizarre subjects. I lost proportion, priorities, and perspective. I was argumentative with my bosses to the extent that I almost lost my job. It affected family life as well. One night I packed all my bags to leave and booked an Uber to JFK [airport]. I went on mood stabilizers, which I still take. It took a long time to find the right one, but it has controlled the manic behavior. MHT didn't help, but because of my poor emotional state I was neglecting my health and didn't use it regularly. One of my friends calls this time of life the "mentalpause."

"I have hot flashes in the classroom"

JENNIFER, FIFTY-ONE, TEACHER, PITTSBURGH

I'm a teacher, and last year my hot flashes were so bad they were interfering with my work. I had a few every hour in front of my nine- and ten-year-old pupils, who were obviously unaware of what was happening—I'd literally just sweat out. It was utterly debilitating. I had three fans around my desk, and I'm overweight, which I know doesn't help. I'd make fun of myself though, and say to them, "Hey guys, this is what happens when you get older."

I'm married with two boys and my sleep was also destroyed, which didn't help the working day. My husband has been incredibly understanding. I've been very open about it, and we're not embarrassed. It's just how my body works. We sleep better by ourselves these days. I need my room, my peace, and a fan.

I'm now on MHT—the patch and a progesterone pill, and that's really helped.

"I lot sweats in the ad world"

ANNA, FIFTY-EIGHT, ADVERTISING BUSINESS OWNER
AND CCO, NEW YORK

Hot flashes have been the most bothersome part of menopause and I used to time them. A minute seems like it lasts forever. My body felt as if I was burning up from the inside out. It's like being that X-Men character who goes from being mild-mannered to burning everything down.

I was doing a lot of presentations whilst deep in the middle of perimenopause. So the hot flashes were frequent and mixed with anxiety of presenting to clients; their onset was pretty severe. Most men were thinking, "*Wow, this woman's sweating a lot in the summer,*" and had no idea what was really happening.

The women's eyebrows raising really bothered me. They made me feel judged. This is when women should support one another. Not judge or demean. Our biology is the same. Eventually every twenty-year-old will stand where I am. And, hopefully with this book, they will find life easier.

CHAPTER NINE

Pretty Menopausal

Cruelly, the menopausal years are when the mental image you have of yourself and the physical reality both start to head south. Declining estrogen can take its toll on face, figure, skin, and hair. You may find yourself, as I did, looking in the mirror and finding that reflection hard to reconcile with the still youthful person bubbling under your wizening visage! I appeared to have been filtered by one of those instant-aging apps, all the rage for snickering at when you're a teen, but becoming far too realistic as you speed toward higher decades! It's a sobering moment to realize that although you still feel (and often act) like the same person you were in your twenties and thirties, the world sees someone markedly different! It's another good reason for trying to build up your store of experience and wisdom to balance the scales. Our attitudes to aging unquestionably need revamping, but one of the heartbreaking discoveries you make as the years speed by is that none of us is actually prepared for the face of "maturity."

I have a theory that we all have an age at which we are fixed in our minds. If you ask friends you'll find that this can vary enormously, some are still shocked they're not eighteen while others can't believe they're not yet seventy! I consider myself lucky that my own sense of myself, and my looks, isn't set back in my early youth, but my late thirties, when my youthful prime was already a topic of nostalgia. Nowadays I sometimes still experience tangible shock waves at the sight of my maturing face. Even with my in-head best-before date set at thirty-eight, it's darkly amusing wondering what my twenty-year-old self would think about what I've become!

Every woman should mature exactly as she pleases without fear of censure or ridicule, but there's no question that a willingness to adapt to changing realities becomes a superpower. Those whimsical floral dresses, that looked so endearing in your twenties and thirties, can become dowdy, and the debate continues to rage about age-appropriate skirt lengths and when to abandon the bikini. On the latter I'm definitely in the Helen Mirren camp—I'm not giving up the two-piece in order to spare the world my post-babies bulge and the shadow of a once proud six pack! Despite the odd loyalty to past favorites, I'd suggest that it's generally unwise to get stuck in a girlish groove that suggests only a dogged determination not to accept your evolution. There's a big difference between looking your best and desperately trying to look twenty years younger. Although maintaining the latter has become the biggest business of the beauty industry, I'm opposed to the whole philosophy of anti- rather than pro-aging; funnily enough there's nothing more aging (and self-destructive) than refusing to accept what you see in the mirror.

It's all very hard work, though. Even base-level glamour from my late forties onwards has required both acceptance and extra maintenance. Hairs start to sprout from unusual places, such as the chin, but become less luxurious on your head. Wrinkles form that seem entirely unrelated to gravity, with pouchy skin forming both below and above your eyes no matter how "clean living" you've become (in my case, not very). Simply staying on top of the day-to-day grooming can be time-consuming at best and an insurmountable challenge at other times.

Increasingly these days there is pressure to hop onto the aesthetic bandwagon, taking your chances with every new treatment available in pursuit of eternal youth. There may be a sweet spot (and of course it's hard to know, as anyone achieving that happy point will look fresh-faced rather than fake), but too often what's achieved is that strange generic look, where you might be anything between forty and seventy. Far easier in the long run to accept the vagaries of time and aim instead to be the best version of ourselves.

That said, how you age is, of course, a natural process and where you draw the line is obviously a personal choice. Sometimes I worry that even plucking my eyebrows is simply succumbing to the patriarchal ideal. On other occasions I wonder how I'd be if I did nothing at all; eyebrows, top lip hair, and beard all coming together as one?

In reality, I suspect that most of us settle for a happy medium, which is what I've tried to do. My hair remains steadfastly blond to public view, I invest in pleasant and efficient face creams, do regular exercise, try to keep my weight steady, and have my irritating frown line Botoxed, but otherwise I allow nature to follow its inexorable course.

Our feelings about our looks around the time of menopause are often at an all-time low, and this negativity can add to the overall sense of struggle. I couldn't find many studies on women and body image in menopause; middle-aged women are the invisible sex in far too many ways, and there's still a societal "who cares" when it comes to analyzing our attempts to remain visibly pleasing. But a 2014 component of SWAN looked at 405 women (39.5 percent Black; 60.5 percent White) aged forty-two to fifty-two and concluded that poor body image may be related to clinically significant depressive symptoms. I'm not sure that required a study, but any investment in tangible research is to be applauded in my book.

"Women with body-image dissatisfaction were more likely to report a clinically significant level of depressive symptoms, as did women who reported feeling unattractive," said the authors. So if you're unhappy with your reflection and feeling pretty down about life, perhaps it's heartening to know that, based on actual science, it's a "thing." You certainly aren't alone, so take hope from that thought.

Professor of health psychology at the UK's University of Surrey, Jane Ogden, is fairly firm on the topic of menopausal self-loathing and looks. Firstly, she reminds us that the aging associated with this time of life is, of course, to some degree inevitable. Consider the alternative: it's better to be alive and looking a bit disheveled than, well, not alive.

"You need to find your sense of identity," she says. "Stop being defined by how you look, and how people react to you. Yes, you may have wrinkles and age spots and your body shape has changed. But your life is written on your face and body. Lines are humor, relationships, and struggles, which, incidentally, define you as much as happiness. Saggy bits might be from having kids or doing a job, which means you can't work out as much as you like. And sun damage is memories of amazing holidays."

I find the concept of wrinkles beautiful because they are the physical story of your adventures both heartening and liberating. As an occasional travel writer and sun worshiper—contravening health, safety, and fashion advice (remember the bikini) every time—I can testify to having my fair share of sun damage. I'd never thought of my face as a grimacing photo album of fun, but It's a more appealing premise than, say, "Your complexion is your karma," which is how I really view my multiple sunspots.

Middle-aged skin also tells the story of your lifestyle, which is possibly less romcom and more psychological thriller in theme if you're low in vital vitamins and minerals and still partying like a sixteen-year-old. It's certainly something I wish I'd been more aware of in my carefree youth, but I'm not sure I would have allowed possible future degradation to mitigate my fun. When you're young, old age seems a universe away, and impossible to imagine. I'd also like to speak up for our more decadent sisters; the more ravaged women I know are often the most fascinating, and certainly the ones you want to hang out with past midnight, on the rare occasions you manage to stay up that late!

I know that when I drink less wine, get more fresh air, glug more water, and sleep better (which often depends on how much alcohol I consume) it's all writ large on my visage. If my face is the book of my life, a couple of days of excess now tell a short story depicted in a pallid complexion and dark circles under my eyes.

Trying too hard to keep change at arm's length is unlikely to yield results, but making sure you are prepped for it is imperative.

We've covered the practicalities of diet and exercise in chapter six, but we need to consider our thinking about food. Eating disorders among the middle-aged are on the rise. "I've been writing about eating behavior and weight management for over thirty years," says Jane. "There's an increase in eating disorders among women in later life; either previous issues returning, or new ones emerging."

Anorexia, bulimia, and binge-eating are by no means solely the remit of teenagers. In 2012, the *International Journal of Eating Disorders* published the results of a study on eating disorders in midlife and beyond. They found that thirteen percent of American women aged fifty or more experienced symptoms. Sixty percent reported that their concerns about weight and shape negatively affected their lives, and seventy percent were trying to lose weight. Furthermore, the highest rates of bulimia plateau around the age of forty-seven—peak perimenopause.

Jane warns that eating disorders can manifest at any time and can be even more damaging in midlife. "Eliminate vital nutrients or consume excess sugar or fat and you won't recover in the same way you might have done in your twenties and thirties," she says. "Plus, you put yourself in serious danger of developing all manner of health conditions including bone loss and damage to your heart and other organs, especially during these years of hormone imbalance. Malnutrition in any form does the menopausal body and mind no favors. Quite genuinely, if you are concerned about your eating, ask for help."

Jane adds that weight-loss injections can be a blessing for those who feel that their weight gain is out of control. "Weight-loss drugs such as Wegovy and Ozempic have given people an additional tool for losing weight without having to go to the extreme and have surgery. Evidence shows that they help with weight loss more than any other drug has done and people feel more in control of their eating behavior and how they look. But," she says (somehow I knew there was going to be a "but"), "we know that when you stop using it the weight tends to go back on, which means that it's likely to be a long-term commitment. In addition, we don't yet know the long-term effects."

Suggesting that social media is the source of all evil hardly qualifies as original thought these days, but unquestionably a great deal of it reaffirms the sense that we need to remain youthful and attractive to maintain our currency. In real life, Jane says that unless you are a model and relying on your looks for actual income, it's unlikely that you are still going to be making friends off the back of "being pretty."

By the time you get to my age there's actually a real sense of liberation to be found in knowing that people aren't spending time with you on the basis of your looks and ability to attract the attention of either sex. They're hanging around because you're interesting, fun, kind, hospitable, adventurous, well-informed, and all the other amazing qualities that you've had a lifetime to develop, and can keep on adding to, despite the dwindling decades in which to pursue them.

When you're young, looks seem paramount, but now, happily, things even out. Those whose popularity and position depended on their superficial attractiveness often struggle most with a sense that their value is diminished (prettiest girl in the school no more). Meanwhile, those who might have focused on developing other attributes find their personalities are now their most seductive attribute. We all get our moment in the spotlight, but some have to wait just a little bit longer for their assets to rise in value.

"Feel better about yourself by making the right comparisons," says Jane. "If you compare yourself to a skincare ad with an 'older' but satin-smooth-skinned model who may be decades younger than you, as well as retouched, then you are going to come off badly. Compare yourself to your peer group, and you'll feel far more cheerful." The ability to zoom in on what you have, rather than what you've lost becomes a superpower. You may have a flabbier tummy (nothing wrong with that, though we all beat ourselves up over it) but you may also have beautiful hair, great legs, or sparklier eyes than those around you of similar age.

Better yet, don't compare. Try to occupy yourself with more holistic goals because if you feel good about yourself, if you are healthy and engaged in life, you'll reflect that positivity into the world around you. It's pleasantly realistic. Don't be afraid to set your own standard. "I didn't wear any makeup through the lockdown months of 2020," says Jane. "It was strange at first, but I soon got used to it. I also think it was good for my students to see me in a state of 'casualness' so they could realize it was OK to just be themselves. Select a norm with which you are happy, not one that others are telling you to embrace, and enjoy it."

There's a brilliantly observed passage in India Knight's novel *Mutton* when her forty-something heroine is so dismayed not to get a reaction from some construction workers she passes that she doubles back to prance past the site again in hope of a more affirming response. Instead, the foreman tips his hard hat and says, "Morning madam." And occasionally it feels cheerfully subversive to look like a younger woman from behind, and then seeing rearview admirers recoil when they realize I'm old enough to be their mother. That famous invisibility of middle age can be dispiriting, but it's also immensely empowering.

Is it really a source of kudos if a stranger thinks we're hot enough to imagine having sex with? Arguably, that's what being physically admired usually comes down to. Going under the radar means that you can sit alone and uninterrupted in a restaurant, enjoying a good book, or have two seats to yourself on a train without some sweaty sleazeball trying to hit on you and ruining your thinking time.

Increasingly, I find myself looking around and appreciating the diversity of beauty in age. All my friends—mostly in their forties upwards—look increasingly attractive as they grow up and into themselves. The years of laughter, the good times and bad emerge on their characterful faces.

There's a brilliantly confrontational scene in the TV series *The Undoing*, when Nicole Kidman's character comes face-to-face with her husband's naked and far younger mistress, even though Nicole has little to worry about on the physical front. Then again, Hollywood actresses seem to be an entirely unique species for whom normal markers of aging, like cellulite and belly pouch, don't exist.

We don't want to leave a stone unturned no matter how "unmentionable" whatever lurks under that rock might be. For example, midlife and beyond is a time during which we might have a rethink about body hair—currently, and bemusingly, deemed repulsively unacceptable among the young. The public changing room where you might be feeling discreetly better about your flabby bits is also one in which you can enjoy the sight of a full bush and feel more relaxed about your grooming. The menopausal years are ones during which hair appears in places it never existed and disappears from others where it's hitherto been taken for granted, and as a friend pointed out recently, whatever your views about the aesthetics, it's not just your face that ages. I know that a million magazine articles say that it's your hands and/or your neck that reveal your true age, but I invite you to examine a fifty- or sixty-year-old vulva and ask friends to place their bets.

It may seem depressing but it's hardly surprising that we begin to feel despondent when mature women are airbrushed from visibility in popular culture, virtually to extinction. We certainly aren't encouraged to think we are looking our best selves when we're all too often absent from advertising, ironically for goods that rely on us as valued consumers. Whether it's movies, TV shows, or media stories about anything other than the trials and indignities of menopause and beyond, we only seem to appear if we've dared to transgress what are considered the norms in terms of expected behavior. I was shocked by the flurry of excitement generated in a newspaper article back in 2017 by my innocently sharing the fact I still love a bikini. You'd think I'd discovered a solution for global warming, or stood up to Vladimir Putin, so venerated was I for a couple of days. UK media was awash with "illustrations" of my "plucky" choice of a two-piece, alongside equally "courageous" abstainers from a full swimming costume, despite a belly showing the telltale signs of past pregnancies and advancing years.

And who hasn't felt a twinge of respect and admiration for such glorious figures as Jerry Hall, stepping out in her swimsuit every summer on the beach next to her house in the South of France, knowing full well that some idiot is lurking in the bushes trying to find a flaw on her sexagenarian supermodel frame so he can make a fast buck. I mean, seriously.

The problem is, if you are not being reflected back an image of yourself that gives you any confidence, it can be extremely hard to muster it when facing the world. I was relieved not to be on the dating market when I hit my fifties, and the outside world confirmed what I was already feeling inside: that my value was plummeting. It may sound superficial, but I doubt it was coincidence that my long-treasured designer discounts from those who had once begged me to wear their fashions, along with my brilliant twenty-year relationship with a top London hairstylist, all ended in that decade. You don't need to be a weatherman to see which way that wind was blowing!

Embracing the physical changes of menopause is about accepting a new version of yourself, no matter how much it's intimated that it's unacceptable. I know that's easier said than done, and especially first thing in the morning when your face looks as though it needs ironing, and it takes until lunchtime for the dent from the eye mask to finally fade. But, if I've gained any wisdom at all, it's not to chase what you can't capture, and youth is something we never stop leaving behind. I very much believe that our menopausal years are those when we have a stronger sense of ourselves. We just need to work on nurturing it.

Whatever steps you decide to take toward teeth whitening, wrinkle fixing, and hair-coloring, don't take it too seriously, and never think that smoother skin or hiding the silver strands is the Holy Grail of contentment. Beauty does not necessarily—and we can all think of extremely sad beauties, both historical and current, old and young—bring happiness. Look around, particularly at real people, not magazine pages and doctored Instagram feeds, and realize that you are doing just fine—it could always be a lot worse. In a decade's time, it actually will be! So, enjoy the moment! We are all constantly evolving and a woman's skill is adapting to new circumstances. Don't think of it as being lesser. Just different. And, in so many ways, more beautiful and interesting.

A Skinful

My face has been put through the wringer over the years. Most of what I ought to have done, I've ignored, and all the basic no-nos, such as "do not bake in direct tropical sun," I've gone ahead and embraced.

Up until the age of fifty, I felt that things were holding together quite nicely, but I noticed a definite drop in smoothness and an increase in pigmentation after that point. There's a sort of blurring around the edges; my once firm jaw is now undulating and my cheeks are less defined. Some days, I think I look like a bad waxwork of myself, as though I have been wafted past a hot flame and melted a little.

"There is chronological aging, and then menopause happens and sort of accelerates some of those natural processes," points out board-certified dermatologist Dr. Lynne Haven. "There's a genetic background that you can't control, but a lot of aging comes from environmental insults," she adds. I love this—I am generally insulted by getting older!

"So, UV light emitted by the sun is a major factor—it creates sunspots, pre-cancerous skin changes, and crepiness," she says. It's a fact that if you compare sun-exposed skin to protected skin there's a massive difference. Look at—for example—your décolletage (always exposed to the sun) and your inner thigh (exposed to the sun for perhaps one week a year) and marvel at how you'd look if you hadn't spent your youth sunbathing.

Pollution is another consideration. "There's blue light from phones and computers, living in a city, those who smoke—if you look at twin studies, the twin who smoked will look older. And then there's also muscle and bone loss to the face. Your jaw shrinks, which contributes to jowls, eye sockets get larger, and teeth shift." These are facts we have to accept or spend our lives doing battle against insurmountable odds.

"Skin color can make a difference to the aging process," she adds. "One reason is that the more melanin you have the less rapidly you tend to develop wrinkles because there's natural protection from sun damage."

Finally, there's collagen loss. This is the protein responsible for skin's structure, elasticity, and that wonderful plumpness of youth. Collagen decreases by about one percent every year from your mid-twenties. "During menopause, levels can plummet by as much as thirty percent in the first five years, which can mean increased dryness and flushing, crepey skin and sagging jowls," says Dr. Haven. As if all this wasn't enough, it's also been shown that menopause is aging us inside and out. In 2016, an American study concluded that menopause speeds up cellular aging by about six percent. Great.

What I've noticed the most is thinning skin, which occurs all over the body, and so it's no surprise to discover that estrogen also has a role in wound healing. Cut a menopausal woman, and she'll bleed for longer . . . In addition, the tip of the nose may sag downward. I came across this fact by accident, but it's true. Your nose, like your boobs and your knees, may droop.

Another incredibly unfair potential menopause side effect is acne, which most of us hoped we'd left behind in puberty and can occur even if you got through your teen years unscathed. Our hormone levels as we know are all over the place, so testosterone might become higher in relation to estrogen, triggering outbreaks of adolescent-like spots.

Rub It In

My mother always told me that, if you look after your face, the rest will take care of itself. Nowadays, it's clear that she was either overly optimistic . . . or lying. Nonetheless, it's advice I took to heart early on, and it's proved a habit that certainly seems to have endured. Despite many shameful debauched nights, I have never, ever, ever gone to bed with my makeup on. I'm not sure it's made any difference to my skin long term, but it certainly allows me to feel smug among my girlfriends, few of whom can claim such an unblemished track record!

I'm also a sucker for good face creams, which have been my greatest investment in luxury throughout life. As I get older, I find I need those that are increasingly rich in texture, as my skin is definitely more Gobi desert than lush tropical rainforest. These days, so manic is my pursuit of moisture that I top up the richest of face creams with a drop of face oil at night. I also try to avoid harmful chemicals, opt for organic products, and use night cream at any point during the day.

So, what expert solutions are available to resolve the aforementioned horrors? Thankfully, plenty. "I tend to break them down into topicals for skin quality and then solutions for the structure of the skin and the face," explains Dr. Haven.

Topically she recommends the golden triangle endorsed by dermatologists and beauty editors worldwide: antioxidants, retinoids, and SPF. "The environment is bombarding your skin with such damaging elements as UV light, smoking, and pollution, so using a vitamin C serum once a day, preferably in the morning, will help neutralize some of these," says Dr. Haven. "Wear SPF year around, and when choosing one, look for those containing titanium dioxide or micronized zinc dioxide—a good-quality active ingredient is more important than the SPF number, and then you might use a mineral-based powder on top, so that you layer the products. Always wear protective clothing, hats, and sunglasses."

I am never happier than when basking near naked in the sun—the world is fortunate that I concede a bikini quite frankly, but that will be why I have wrinkles all over my body and I'd bet that Dr. Haven doesn't.

Then there are retinoids, which are forms of vitamin A that work on skin to exfoliate and increase cell turnover, so it looks revitalized. "They can be helpful for a wide range of concerns, from acne to sun damage. You need to find one that's tolerable to your skin, as there can be redness and sensitivity. Some of the newer formulas are micronized or time release, and therefore less irritating. Always wear SPF with retinoids as they repair sun damage, but they also make you more sun sensitive."

You will probably want to use a serum or moisturizer along with this trio. Relatively new to the world of anti-aging are phytoestrogen products. "These contain a synthetic or plant-derived estrogen that attaches to the estrogen receptors in skin and can rejuvenate the menopausal complexion." Other topical products are growth factors, which stimulate skin cell turnover. "As we age, cells renew themselves less frequently." Or you might choose something containing hyaluronic acid to moisturize that dry mature skin. "I also like topicals with ceramides, which are naturally moisturizing, and can be depleted in aging skin."

I was hesitant about including a how-to of aesthetic treatments. I know a lot of women who have a syringe of Botox or a facial peel to look brighter and feel better. But equally, I know just as many who feel that they are quite beautiful enough and would rather go on vacation or buy a new car.

In the spirit of full confession, I've had twice-annual Botox for the deep frown lines I'm prone to between my brows, the legacy of a lifetime as a bookworm. I have also had a treatment called the Six Point Lift, conducted by a charming Frenchman called Dr. Dray, which involved injecting hyaluronic acid into six points on my face. I think it assisted in the tussle with wrinkles, but no one ever commented on it, so the benefits were clearly subtle!

"There are many solutions, most of which we'd offer for normal aging, rather than menopause specifically," says Dr. Haven. "Lasers are very beneficial for skin tightening and resurfacing to help with the signs of sun damage, wrinkling, and building collagen and elastin. A lot of women during this time will have increased redness and sensitivity as well as acne, for which we have a whole host of traditional acne medicines.

"In terms of skin structure, there are many fillers that can be used to resculpt the face, and hyaluronic acid fillers that can be used as skin boosts—adding moisture back into the face."

Don't be a guinea pig, don't go cheap, and don't, for goodness' sake, buy Botox on the internet and try to inject it yourself. This was a ridiculous trend a few years ago, and a browse on Google confirms that, yes, you can still do so. No good can ever come of this.

Grit Your Teeth

If you are prone to the classic anxiety dream where all your teeth fall out, then stop reading now. Who knew that the mouth was affected by menopause? I certainly didn't, although I am meticulous about attending dental appointments. However, just like the vagina, the mouth needs lubrication. "Estrogen affects every part of your body, and that includes the mouth," says board-certified periodontist Dr. Leena Palomo, professor and chair of the Ashman Department of Periodontology and Implant Dentistry at New York University, College of Dentistry. "Changes in blood supply affect the salivary organs and the soft tissues of the mouth. Salivary glands produce either less saliva or a different mixture of fluids and salts, so mouths become drier. This can be linked to discomfort, yeast infection, and those pesky little cracks that you get at the corner of your mouth—especially in winter." We are, she says, dry on the outside and dry on the inside, and dry mouth is linked to tooth decay.

"Gum disease can get much worse during menopause, but this isn't directly because of dry mouth. When we think about periodontal disease, we think about the pink gums. But under these is that bony socket. Some research suggests that there's a greater susceptibility to reabsorption of that bone during menopause. Bacteria in the mouth in a non-menopausal and therefore less susceptible patient might not be a problem, but it might be a greater problem in a menopause patient." There is a higher incidence of tooth loss in menopausal patients, she adds.

That lack of saliva swishing around the teeth also means that you're more likely to see staining; we all know about the potential damage from coffee, tea, and red wine, but even herbal tea can give teeth a bit of a brown tinge. I have personal experience with the aging mouth and all the joys it brings. Aged fifty, I noticed that all my lower teeth were caving inwards and went rushing off to an orthodontist, who suggested Invisalign—clear, fitted braces. Better than a facelift, he said, for looking youthful; teeth are vital in maintaining the structure of your face. Two years later, they certainly looked better, but then I discovered that there is no "afterward," and I had to add a nightly retainer to my ever-expanding bedtime routine. I wonder how long I'll manage to keep up the level of maintenance. It's not the most come-hither look to be flashing a plastic tooth cover (along with eye mask and silicone ear plugs) as you settle back on the pillows in your vintage satin.

Dr. Palomo sees a lot of women around the age of menopause who've never had any problems with their mouths, but suddenly find that things are shifting or uncomfortable. "In order to support a tooth that bony socket needs to be high around the necks of teeth," she says. "If it is reabsorbed, chewing can become a problem—and the first food to go is protein as we turn to softer foods—carbohydrates such as bread and cakes, which is terrible for blood sugar, and especially during menopause. We grind our teeth if we're upset and if they are less supported, they might migrate." Once teeth don't fit together anymore, we can have a clicking and painful jaw as well as cosmetic problems. Grinding teeth can also lead to muscle pain and headaches.

My teeth-grinding during stressful insomniac nights has actually cracked one of my lower molars, which now has to go. The cliché of the toothless crone draws ever closer.

Some women also get what's called burning mouth syndrome, which isn't cosmetically displeasing, but can be quite distressing—a sort of "burning" pain. "Burning mouth can also be a symptom of something called erosive lichen planus," says Dr. Palomo. "This can become malignant, so you need to be aware of it."

The biggest problem is the fear of losing teeth—let's face it, we've all gone to the dentist occasionally feeling sheepish and terrified. But what I find reassuring is that Dr. Palomo says it's never too late to fix teeth, or their appearance. "At the end of the day it's about quality of life. It's about aesthetics and it's about function in terms of biting into food and chewing or function in terms of comfort.

"For generations, women have been told that their pain is imaginary. We need to be vigilant and speak up when something isn't right." We also, she says, need to be a part of the solution. "As well as reporting what's happening, we need to remember that what our mothers told us is still true. Brush teeth for two minutes twice a day and floss. Nobody likes to floss, but it's necessary. Visit the dentist at least twice a year—for those with problems this might need to be four times." For burning mouth, use alcohol-free mouthwash, which is less irritating, as well as SLS (sodium lauryl sulfate)-free toothpaste, avoid alcohol and acidic foods, and give up smoking. "I like toothbrushes which link to apps as they ensure you don't miss any little areas of the mouth."

A 2017 study showed that MHT appeared to make a difference (I promise, I'm not on commission): rates of gum disease were lower in those taking it. "It can be good for lubrication," concedes Dr. Palomo. "But increase of blood flow in the presence of plaque can mean more, not less, inflammation."

I asked about teeth whitening—you Americans are famous for your excellent white teeth (we Brits are also famous for our teeth, but for less favorable reasons), and there's no question that a straight white smile makes you look far healthier (OK, and younger). Dr. Palomo says there's huge demand for aesthetic support from midlife women. "Enamel ages because of what it's exposed to, such as coffee and red wine, but when you think about whitening, it's about the hue and also the opacity of the teeth." She says that if you want to go a few shades lighter then there are over-the-counter products. "But think about the entire aesthetic—the shape, size, and alignment of the teeth, how the lip-line looks on the teeth, and should you wish for more then see a specialist."

And should you or your teeth need more serious support, there are a variety of ways in which they can be helped—dental implants, advanced bone grafting, tissue grafting. "You don't need to look long in the tooth anymore. Just always make sure you tell your dentist of any concerns. Think of your teeth as being a story. Our bodies change, our bones change, and our teeth change. Looking after them is like an arc not a set point in time."

Heavy Is the Head (of Hair)

My hair history is a saga in itself: three early decades of trauma, followed by twenty years during which time my glossy blond bob was described as my "trademark." It's always a bit disappointing to hear that any thought or idea I've aired over nearly six decades is nothing compared to the effect achieved by two hours in the Mayfair salon that I visited from my mid-thirties to mid-fifties.

I became entirely dependent on good hair, my confidence in any presenting job or public appearance reliant on whether I could squeeze in a blow-dry beforehand. As I passed the mid-forties mark, I noticed that well-groomed hair was the perfect foil for a host of other "imperfections"—tired skin or dark circles under the eyes, for example—and it became the number one priority of my beauty regimen.

I have always had fine hair, as well as zero skills with beauty tools, whether attempting a blow-dry or a DIY manicure. In unkempt youth, hair that looks as though you've just crawled from a tussle between the sheets is sexy. When you're in your fifties, it's not the first image you want people to conjure up. In the last decade, I've noticed that the length can't go past my jaw without looking messy.

But my own adventures aside, it turns out that, just like the rest of the body, hair ages, and of course menopause can have an impact.

"Some women barely notice a difference around the time of menopause, but others will see noticeable thinning, which can be incredibly distressing psychologically," says Anabel Kingsley, leading New York–based consultant trichologist and brand president of the Philip Kingsley Clinics. "Women feel they are losing their identity and femininity."

And hair can hugely affect mood. Dr. Marianne LaFrance at Yale University worked with Pantene for two decades, and a 2017 global study she conducted concluded that a great hair day makes women feel strong, and was also associated with feeling "more productive, less stressed, more socially powerful, more resilient, physically stronger, and more in control." That's a lot of pressure on our hair! "The women who come to see me at menopause feel that their identity is being challenged in a number of ways," agrees Anabel.

There are two reasons why hair may become a concern at this time of life. Firstly, the normal growth phase of hair lasts between three and seven years, and this is maintained by estrogen. "A big drop in estrogen around menopause shortens the growth phase and leads to more shedding of hair." We all lose around eighty to one hundred hairs every single day, but around the age of fifty, many women notice increased hair loss and seek help. When hormone turbulence settles down this is likely to return to the normal range.

In addition, as estrogen goes down, testosterone can become more dominant. Many of us have hair follicles—the bulb in the scalp from which the hair grows—which are sensitive to testosterone levels. "In those with a genetic predisposition, follicles may become smaller and hair won't be as long or thick, with a shorter growth cycle.

"This is what's known as androgenetic alopecia, or female-pattern hair loss, and is very common among women. Where men go bald, women usually see a more diffuse thinning around the head and parting," says Anabel. It's a gradual process, and you will probably lose around twenty percent of the density before noticing. It is said to affect up to forty percent of women by the age of fifty—Anabel thinks most women experience a little thinning during these years. "There are other subtle differences. Hair becomes finer as scalp and hair-cell quality ages along with the rest of the body. Do not panic. You may not even notice."

"It's a good idea to seek help as soon as you notice thinning hair," says Anabel. "A good trichologist can promise maintenance of density and can often improve severe thinning, but it's not always possible to completely restore." You can obtain prescription scalp drops containing both minoxidil and estradiol benzoate—which is topical estrogen. MHT—replenishing estrogen levels—can certainly help as well.

"We support a lot of clients who have suffered hair loss through breast cancer treatment (and always write to their oncologist if relevant to do so)." You might also try minoxidil (which you can buy over the counter as Rogaine for Women) on its own, which is the hair-growth scalp treatment with FDA approval (basically the gold star tried-and-tested) and is the most effective hair-growth formula for women. The only problem with minoxidil is that you have to keep using it.

Low iron and ferritin levels are also associated with thinning hair. If periods are lighter or have stopped, then this is less likely to be a problem, but if you are one of those whose periods have become heavier, then remember that the last part of your body to receive vital nourishment is always your hair. This is why fad diets are likely to affect hair growth.

Every hair follicle has a vitamin D receptor, so low levels of this can affect hair health. Anabel sees a lot of vitamin D deficiency, especially in those of us over forty who are—too late for me—aware of sun damage.

It's easier said than done, especially if every day is a bad hair day, but try to keep stress levels down. As Anabel explains: "Stress raises testosterone levels and creates imbalance, as well as impacting your scalp's microflora and how your gut absorbs vital nutrients, which can create problems for the hair and scalp."

Color Me Radiant

As for my hair color, which has defined me for much of my career, these days it's faker than ever! For historical context, I developed my own badger's white stripe across my parting almost overnight, at the age of fifteen, when my father died. Back then, it was mortifying to have this blast of white hair in what I dimly recall as being a basic mousy brown. Besides, it was the 1970s, and thanks to the original Blondie herself, and also Sid Vicious of the Sex Pistols, bleach blond was all the rage—the less realistic the better. I've been dyeing mine lighter ever since and it's been so long that I can't truly remember the original color (though when I look at my daughter's tumbling locks of auburn honey–coated gorgeousness, I know the hues didn't come from me). Now I suspect if I let it grow out it would be pure white, which I'm thinking is the way to go to celebrate my next big birthday. But they do say that blondes have more fun, and as you get older you don't want to short-change yourself, so I might hang on in there.

As if in answer to my ponderings, Josh Wood, world-leading celebrity colorist whose clients include Australian singer and actress Kylie Minogue and Australian model Elle Macpherson, says that you don't have to do a drastic overhaul. "As you age, and skin color changes, think of your hairline as being a frame for your face. The color around here needs to be a little softer and lighter, no matter what your hair type. It's all about complementing skin tone.

"Color is a great way to make hair look thicker, especially around the parting," he adds. "Loss of pigment means that the scalp can be more evident; it's more apparent in darker hair."

Color can also create the illusion of thicker hair all over the head. "The more contrast between light and dark, the more you give the illusion of thickness. You need to keep it multidimensional, with lots of different color strands, and using techniques such as highlights, balayage, and root tints."

For those of you who like a semi-permanent color, increased scalp sweating might mean considering permanent color, and if you have any dye touching the scalp, have a patch test every time. "For some reason, this is a time when you may suddenly develop an allergy or an irritation to certain products, and this can cause breakouts around the nape of the neck."

Makeup

There was a watershed moment in my early fifties when I realized that makeup had become compulsory unless I was in strict hibernation. Being barefaced no longer suggested fresh and healthy but gave me the look of Victorian late-stage consumption. A tinted moisturizer is now compulsory until mid-summer, when I let my natural tan take over. Plenty of women still look amazing barefaced and I'm consumed with envy for their natural beauty. My problem was that I'd started to lose my eyes, and with my lopsided, asymmetrical face, that was unfortunate. They'd always been the feature I'd zoomed in on (long before actual Zoom, of course), but now, without a little accentuation, they were barely an asset. First thing in the morning, my makeup-free face can look as flat and as dull as a cloudy November morning.

So the luxury of greeting the world fully makeup free is not the best option for me. To mitigate, I never leave the house without a daube of Bobbi Browns Taupe Eye Crayon (a lovely caramel) eyeshadow on my lids, and for evenings, hallelujah for Victoria Beckham's genius EyeWear Shadow Sticks, creamy and in delectable shades for a bit of nighttime drama. I have a semi-regular dedication to dyed eyebrows and lashes, which lifts my whole face. I love Benefit's Benetint Lip and Cheek Stain, which gives your cheeks that soft flush of youthful excitement—which obviously needs faking these days, and Trinny's BFF Skin Perfector covers imperfections and adds a fresh glow.

I can see exactly why makeup artists like Bobbi Brown with her Jones Road line, or Charlotte Tilbury's cosmetics, have become so phenomenally successful. Everything they produce creates luminosity, and that's in short supply over the age of fifty, even with a Gwyneth Paltrow–level healthy lifestyle. And if you can buy it from Tilbury, why suffer the deprivations needed for superhuman health obsessions!

It transpires that I am neither unique nor alone with my mysteriously disappearing features. "From about fifty-five, there's a noticeable fading of features on the face, and the paler the skin, the more evident this is," says Tricia Cusden, the trailblazing beauty vlogger who founded makeup brand Look Fabulous Forever out of frustration at the lack of advice and makeup for older women. Her YouTube tutorials have received well over five million views.

"We call this the loss of luminance of contrast. In a younger face, you can clearly see the definition of eyes, lips, cheeks, and eyebrows. But after menopause it's not so obvious. The great thing about makeup is that you can use it to restore both color and definition."

I can confirm that I have lost my luminance of contrast, and am happy to take more tips on board. I asked legendary makeup artist Sandy Linter, whose clients include Elizabeth Hurley and Christie Brinkley, for advice. "It's important mentally to like what we see in the mirror. It gives us energy. I took the less natural way to age—I think because I was in the fashion industry and surrounded by many who could recommend a top-notch surgeon." But she adds, you should always appreciate yourself. "I'm seventy-six now, and fifty looks young to me. Please take it from me, you look younger than you think you do!"

Incidentally, the look I think we're all trying to avoid, but one that we risk as our sight gets worse, is that slightly crazed caked-on look, with lipstick seeping into the lines around our mouths and wonky black eyeliner.

That said, I wonder whether we ought to be looking for a foundation that offers more coverage—house paint, perhaps? No, says Sandy. Quite the opposite. "I think the reverse is true. I know a lot of people think you can cover age spots and wrinkles with heavy foundation, but the weird thing about makeup is that as you get older less and lighter is better. You cannot conceal wrinkles—just keep that area lightly made up. Go half a shade warmer than your natural skin tone and make sure you blend foundation around the neck with a brush. Dab concealer onto sunspots or areas you want to cover up, and you need a little brush to apply it. Fingers have a little heat in them, and you'll struggle to keep the product on your face."

If you are suffering from hot flashes, she recommends using a primer on top of your moisturizer. "Otherwise, you might find your foundation dripping off your face." For dark circles—the curse of the insomniac menopausal woman—she says to keep concealer along the groove of the circle and blend it in. "The biggest mistake is choosing a color that's too light. If you can see the concealer, you need to go half a shade deeper."

Eyes are my focus more than lips, and Sandy recommends using fake lashes for the sparse remains of my once lustrous lashes. "If you are using strip ones, cut them into three sections. Apply from the ends and work inwards. Otherwise get a great lash curler and mascara, and only ever do two coats." If your brows are thinning, she suggests using a brow serum that contains peptides, or semi-permanent coloring.

So, there in a nutshell is a mixture of my personal experience, lessons learned the hard way, and the expert advice of specialists in the beauty field. In many ways this is the trickiest topic to cover thanks to my resentment that the acceptability bar for mitigating the impact of aging seems set ludicrously and unfairly high for women. One of the things that gives me comfort, and a sense of purpose to continue my efforts to enhance what I still have, is how much worse the majority of men look in their later years. The world can laugh at us for our vanity and superficiality in our pursuit of longer-lasting looks, and outlay on products promising us minor miracles, but put a well-groomed woman in her seventies and a man the same age who's never used a beauty product in his life in front of a judging panel and I know who'll get the gold star . . .

"I am kinder to myself now"

BESTSELLING AUTHOR MARIAN KEYES, SIXTIES, DUBLIN

I never felt that I fit the template of a sexy and attractive woman. I've always been the person who is ignored in the queue in the shop. I'm short and I have a meek face. Shopkeepers look at me and they think,

"She'll be no trouble. I'm going to deal with the trickier people first." So, in some ways, and this is going to sound weird, but I feel more attractive now than I did in my twenties. I suppose I was probably much more objectively attractive then, but I hated myself so much and I self-sabotaged all the time, so it was no good with me. Now, I'm in my sixties, and I know I scrub up well. I am kinder to myself now. Partly it's because I'm more confident, better able to stand up for myself and carve out my place in a conversation.

I feel happier in myself. I don't think of myself just as looks. I know that I tend to be kind. I'll go out of my way to make people feel comfortable, that my looks are part of a package of a decent person.

And I don't know what you can make of this, but I take a huge amount of care of my appearance now. I have Botox, I have fillers, and I care about my skin. It matters to me. I think because of that I don't feel less visible now, which is nice.

When you're younger, you have this idea that looks are everything. When you're older, people aren't drawn to you by beauty alone. We want more. If you're not kind or entertaining or clever, or if you aren't present, it doesn't matter how physically beautiful you are.

"I've hated my hair loss"

EMILY, FIFTY-TWO, NUTRITIONAL COUNSELOR, SAN FRANCISCO

I'm healthy, and exercise a lot, so I'm kind of a boring person. But the worst menopause symptom has been hair loss. I'm still getting my period, but since October 2023 I've lost clumps every time I wash it. I've always been proud of my hair, and watching it swirling down the drain was horrible. I felt as though I was losing my sense of self, and very rapidly I could see my scalp showing white beneath. I started using a hair supplement but it didn't make any difference, and then tried oral minoxidil, which is slowing it down, as well as other supplements, a hair serum, and special shampoo, but

I'm not seeing any regrowth yet. It has been and continues to be an extremely stressful thing to worry about, and not something I was expecting in my perimenopausal years.

"I was terrible during menopause"

ALICIA COPPOLA, FIFTY-FIVE, ACTRESS AND DIRECTOR, LOS ANGELES

I kind of feel like being a woman of fifty-five I have so much more to offer than I ever did. But it's a harder sell than it was in my twenties or thirties. Ageism is alive and well, and the roles I'm offered have certainly been affected. They aren't as plentiful and therefore harder to come by. I consider myself very viable and I think I'm aging well. As the model Paulina Porizkova coined . . . I am somewhere between J-Lo and Betty White!

LA is the land of keep it tight, keep it skinny, and keep it young, especially in the business of acting. I think I am only getting better. But after you get to forty it's harder.

During my menopause I was a terrible cunt. I was really un-friendly, and snappy. I've always dealt with anxiety and depression, and I've always had stomach issues, but they got worse. My period had always been pretty consistent but that changed. Then I started to have trouble sleeping and focusing. I have had hot flashes at work, whilst under the hot lights. I had to mention it to the director of photography, who is a wonderful man. He was like "We got you," and they brought in fans and stuff. It happened three times. I now travel with those packs that you punch and they become ice cold—just in case.

Now I think I'm done. But I do have this lovely thing called the meno belly. Like *what*? Nobody told me that all of a sudden I'm gonna look like I'm three months pregnant all the time. I'm skinny everywhere else. I have a tall frame. And now I have this paunch! It won't exercise away. The indignities!

However, I'm creating and hustling, and I have more energy for that than when I was younger. I go where the day takes me because the day is all we are given, so I want to make the most of it. I've written and directed two short films. *Between Us* and *And You Are . . . ?* starring a fellow Brit, the incomparable Jane Seymour! I'm looking to enhance my career as a director by using my thirty-plus years of being an actress and being on set. My education is phenomenal and I am super proud of the work I have been given and the work I have created and have yet to create!

"Injections held off my weight gain"

ANASTASIA, FIFTY, CEO, CONNECTICUT

In my late forties I gained about forty pounds. No matter how much exercise I did, I was unable to lose it, and it was very depressing. So I decided to try the GLP-1 injections to see what happened. They were incredible. I was prescribed them by my doctor, and it was as though a switch had been pressed on the chatter in my head about food. I hadn't realized that it was a constant voice, but losing that gave me the bandwidth to do so much more, as well as losing the weight. But you have to stay on it to maintain the weight loss, and now it's incredibly hard to get hold of—it's out of stock and I've been calling round pharmacies to track it down.

CHAPTER TEN

Hot Sex

There's a strange disconnect when it comes to older women and sex. Studies show that we're saying yes yes yes well into our nineties, so you'd think the conversation about sex would be central to the menopausal gold rush that's defining the 2020s. But acknowledging that you might want sex in your sixties and beyond is seemingly still a social taboo outside your close friendship circle. Sex as the preserve of youth is what the world reflects to us, whether in advertising or influencer stories, so it's easy to feel as though that's the true narrative. Teenagers might eagerly exchange details about a first kiss, but shouting from the rooftops about an octogenarian orgasm is societally far less welcome. What's acceptable isn't necessarily reflective of the reality, and like so much else in the midlife conversation, mature sex is slowly emerging as big business. Cosmopolitan.com recently did a digital issue entitled "Sex After 60," packed with information about sex toys, the lack of a female Viagra (Where's *our* Little Blue Pill?), and awash with quotes from older women about the joys of sex in your seventh decade and beyond.

As a baby boomer, I'm used to discriminatory attitudes toward women's sex organs. Having grown up during those dark ages when men used to shudder at the very mention of that fishy-smelling no-go zone worthy of penetration only, it's still a pinch-me moment to find myself in an era when Gwyneth Paltrow's This Smells Like My Vagina candle was a bestseller. Though it's depressing to see that its sister candle is entitled Hands Off My Vagina—a reference to *Roe vs Wade* being overturned.

The main reason I accepted a role in *The Vagina Monologues* in 2001, aside from my co-stars (I was totally obscured by the brilliance of my two partners: actresses Marianne Jean-Baptiste and Amy Irving), was because of the subversive delight in saying the words "vagina" and "cunt" a hundred times a night, in celebration rather than trepidation. Image improvements aside, it's a body part that generally misses out on the self-care we give our faces, hands, and feet, and other than being the hotspot for sexual pleasure, unless we're pregnant or have an STD, it tends to barely feature in our maintenance schedule. That all needs to change in middle age, when scenting or waxing are barely grazing the spot, so to speak.

It's not just the more commonly publicized difficulties that can present, like vaginal dryness, an endless propensity to pee, and recurring urinary tract infections, but also thinning pubic hair and, rather upsettingly, it's not just the top of your head that goes gray! The day I found my first gray pube, I seriously considered booking my slot at Dignitas—the assisted suicide clinic. It's a sad day when you fall into deep mourning for your once lustrous, gleaming pubic hair!

With perfect synchronicity, the day I sat down to write this chapter the doorbell rang and I was presented with a gift box brimming with items specifically for the vagina and vulva (and no, they weren't from an ex-lover or my current husband!). Within, I discovered an entirely new world, devoted to the most personal of beauty ranges: a daily intimate wash, an intimate calming oil, various other scented lovelies, and a lollipop shaped like a vulva, which, having been on a sugar-free diet for two weeks, I immediately ate.

Skincare for our sex organs may seem a step too far on the to-do list for a generation of women already juggling responsibilities like circus professionals, and I'm inherently suspicious of any routine devoted to wiping out my natural odor (although, if Annick Goutal did an Eau d'Hadrien vaginal spray, I might be tempted to take my perfume lower than my neck). Remembering to cleanse, tone, and moisturize my face every day is hard enough, so adding further chores isn't an option unless they're essential.

But there are items that are well worth including in your bedside drawer. The good news is, with a little bit of concentration, an embracing of the inevitable, and the determination to maintain a manageable self-care routine, it doesn't need to be the end of the world for your body below the waist! But you can't just lie back and think of England (or New York). It appears that these just might be necessary new to-dos, and these days, I liberally and routinely apply moisturizer to anywhere that requires it.

The Bare Facts

What we aren't told about changes to our vaginas from our forties on-wards is another shocking example of the veil of silence around women's health. The vagina isn't just an area for sexual play and baby-making, but a vital part of the reproductive system that sits among a cluster of nearby organs where loss of estrogen takes its toll. It's important for both making babies, and getting them out, along with a great deal of entertainment and hospitality.

As for "nit-picking" between vagina and vulva (OK, OK, I know they're anatomically different), if, like me, you're a late-comer to the differences, let's summarize the areas of concern: the vagina is the muscular canal with the cervix at the top. If you're heading upwards, it's where sperm travels to find the egg, and, going down, it connects the uterus to the outside world, so that babies and menstrual blood can come out. It's around three inches long but is, of course, super stretchy.

The outside bit is the vulva, which includes the labia (inner and outer), the clitoris, and vaginal and urethral openings (where the pee comes out). Like the rest of the body, the vulva and vagina alter with age, and never more so than at this time of hormonal flux.

Issues with the vagina or vulva don't tend to score top billing on lists of symptoms, playing second fiddle to the flashier and certainly more obvi-ous, hot flash. It's almost as though the general assumption is that older women shouldn't be having sex, and it's certainly not worth keeping our-selves booty-call prepared. Don't get me wrong, discussing it as frankly as I am here raises a blush, and has involved some heated internal debate, but my desire to bust the cycle of shame has overridden any sense of decorum I'd hoped to maintain.

As we know, estrogen controls lubrication; dry mouth and dry eyes are common as it declines. But it's also essential for the health and comfort of the bladder, vagina, and vulva. Take away natural hydration, add in thin-ning skin, alter the pH levels, remove the muscle tone, and you're poten-tially facing all manner of problems.

There can be dryness, itching, soreness, and pain during intercourse and urinating. The wall of the urethra, the duct that carries urine from the bladder, becomes thinner and more sensitive, the pelvic-floor muscle loses tone, which can mean leaking urine, and there's an increased likelihood of urinary tract infections (UTIs) and thrush. The vagina becomes shorter, tighter, and the skin less elastic.

This all comes together in a rather unspeakable phrase: genitourinary syndrome of menopause (GSM). Makes you shiver with horror, no? It is also called vaginal atrophy (and most often googled as vaginal dryness), which is no less unpleasant in connotation, but slightly more usefully descriptive. Problems tend to manifest later in the menopausal transition and beyond, but can start as early as your forties—perhaps with discomfort during a Pap smear. There is no way of knowing how many women actually suffer, because most endure what can be genuinely torturous symptoms in silence and don't dare seek medical advice. Very few of us, myself included, particularly want to confide in our doctors and endure the possible embarrassment of a face-to-face or, I suppose, a vulva to face, experience.

"Vaginal changes tend to occur later in the menopausal transition. They don't resolve without treatment, and are likely to get worse," says Dr. Mary Jane Minkin. "Bladder symptoms in particular must not be ignored," she emphasizes. "In far older women a UTI can lead to urosepsis and even death." She currently has an eighty-year-old patient who is suffering from recurrent UTIs, but is struggling to get the right vaginal estrogen approved by her insurance company. "She's a nun, and not sexually active, so she can't get the applicator inside her vagina and needs a type with a far smaller applicator. I was on the phone for an hour explaining that without it she could get seriously unwell."

Studies offer clues to prevalence, but there's little consensus; some say fifty percent of women and others seventy percent (e.g., nobody actually knows). I'd say—based on nothing but a knowledge of the embarrassment around the subject (certainly no medical expertise!)—that it's probably more like one hundred percent. Most importantly, the majority of women aren't seeking help. When I found myself regularly getting a UTI on the dwindling occasions my husband and I managed to squeeze intercourse onto our to-do list, I was puzzled. Surely this is a condition synonymous with carefree youthful coupling, when you'd be at it all night, and wind up suffering for your enthusiasm with a bath in baking soda to ease the burning.

I had no idea that, for entirely different, and far less erotic, reasons, even routine love making of swift duration could induce similar agonies; the urethra is more likely to get infected if you're lacking moisture, and also because of the thinning skin and a change in the local bacteria.

After a few months of this debilitating condition recurring, I slipped it in as a seemingly inconsequential last-minute query at a routine doctor's appointment, hand already on the door to leave. Luckily, I was in the presence of a pro and far from increasing my evident discomfort, I was advised that urinating within fifteen minutes of having sex can wash away the bacteria and save menopausal midlifers from the all-too-common symptoms of cystitis. Other treatments recommended included being well hydrated, using over-the-counter painkillers, and—if needed—antibiotics. But there was never a mention of vaginal estrogen—a treatment that is proven to work. Incidentally, Dr. Minkin says that cranberry products can also be effective against developing UTIs.

As my story proves, staying silent is not the answer. I subsequently only had the odd bout of cystitis, but it was a glimpse into the world of a quite extraordinary lady I came across, called Jane Lewis. She suffered from seriously debilitating vaginal atrophy for seven years, from her early forties, and wrote the compelling—I mean this, it's hilarious—book called *Me and My Menopausal Vagina*, with her daughter.

"Women aren't seeking help for vaginal atrophy symptoms, and by not doing so they are perpetuating the feelings of secrecy and shame," says Jane. Vaginal atrophy can, she says, destroy your quality of life. "It's the forgotten symptom and, quite genuinely, a sore subject."

She describes her experience thus: "Imagine if you had a really dry mouth, but couldn't drink anything, so it splits and cracks and bleeds and burns. You'd be aware of it every second of the day." Jane recounts being unable even to sit down because of the burning pain, and using cans of frozen baked beans wrapped in a towel to press against her nether regions to temporarily alleviate the agony. To me, this undignified solution is reminiscent of childbirth—you get to a point where you simply don't care what happens, so long as the pain stops.

The idea of seven years of (well-documented) suffering is eye-opening. In spite of having the most extraordinarily supportive family, she was in such distress that she considered taking her own life. "One day, my daughter called up and kept me on the phone for ages. I thought she was at work, but then she arrived on my doorstep. She says that she was worried I might harm myself."

Did she have sex during this time? "What do you think? For some women, sex becomes painful, so they stop having it entirely. Then the pain goes, but this means the area is completely unused. Pelvic exams become impossible, or you may get repeated UTIs [which chimes with my own experience], and then the whole vulva area becomes sore, itchy, and burns when you wee.

"My experience sounds dramatic, but it's certainly not rare," she says. "Women put up with things and self-treat, but it's not necessary." Perhaps you are reading this and nodding a little bit, even grimacing, in recognition, and realizing that repeated UTIs is not normal, or that painful sex might have a solution. Have a chat with your doctor.

Jane is now—you will be relieved to hear—in a far better place, relatively speaking, but she reminds me that this is for life.

"I still can't wear skinny jeans, I'll never ride a horse again, but I can sit in the cinema. I have a routine: I wash twice a day with water, and I apply moisturizer. You aren't suddenly going to start producing more estrogen. If you need local estrogen—one of the most effective treatments (as a gel, pessary, or ring)—that's going to be forever; don't be fobbed off with a short course. And don't let anyone tell you that you can't take systemic MHT and use local estrogen. Yes, you can."

In addition to many of us not discussing our private parts (centuries of body shaming will do that), there are still blinkered views about sexuality. Also there are communities and individuals who struggle to speak about sex, which makes it harder to find solutions where there are difficulties. "I think this is cultural," says Omisade Burney-Scott, founder of Black Girl's Guide to Surviving Menopause. "It's how people have been raised in terms of understanding their sexuality, and the recognition that there's a spectrum of sexuality. In Black communities there's been a growing movement to help people unlearn the stereotypes and tropes about what Black sexuality and intimacy looks like. And there's been a lot of work to help people understand that pleasure is not always synonymous with sexual intercourse. And there's a lot of assumptions about heteronormativity where we think that everybody's experience is heterosexual or that they gender identify as a woman."

Tending Your Lady Garden

In my day, we used to snicker about K-Y Jelly, but as you reach maturity, one of the new generation of sexual lubricants without harmful chemicals (no one should be shoving anything with the potential for irritation into their most intimate parts) is not just a bottom-drawer aid to kinkier diversions, but essential for routine coupling. Yes, your bedside table needs to contain a tube of lube. But it's not that simple.

Googling "lube" offers a baffling array of products. It's truly a sight for all the sore parts. There's plain, there's silky, sensual, strawberry, and there's sensitive. What a world. The temptation is to either swear off sex for the rest of your life or pop the first product you see into your basket.

Lubrication may be the secret to postmenopausal sex for the majority of women, but which is right for me?

"Most people like to try over-the-counter solutions first as they're cheaper and you don't have to be in contact with a physician," says Dr. Minkin. "Just remember that vaginal tissue is the most sensitive in the body, so avoid perfumed products as well as potentially irritating ingredients such as glycerin."

Many need more than basic lubrication and there are moisturizers, available from drugstores, that can be placed in the vagina every day. "If you also have urinary symptoms, or this isn't sufficient, then vaginal estrogens are FDA approved, safe for use if you've had breast cancer, and they can also be used alongside systemic estrogen in women who have not had breast cancer," says Dr. Minkin. "These come in several forms; creams, tablets, and rings; the creams can be used both internally and externally. You can insert the cream with a plunger or use fingers both inside the vagina and around the vulva externally. Tablets come with an applicator to be used daily, usually for two weeks, and then twice a week, and the ring is a soft rubber ring that looks like a diaphragm without the cup." Ninety-nine percent of users don't notice this, she says. "There's also a new oral medication available called ospemifene, which is what's called a SERM (selective estrogen receptor modulator) and improves vaginal moisture as well as bladder symptoms." This is not an estrogen and is appropriate for breast cancer survivors.

It's worth pointing out that vaginal estrogen boxes come with the same information as systemic estrogens, and the same dire (and incorrect) breast cancer warnings, which means that, should they read it, patients might be scared to use it. "The Menopause Society has gone to the FDA and asked that they be removed," says Dr. Minkin. "A very small amount of estrogen is absorbed and there is no breast cancer risk."

Should sex be painful, in addition to lubrication, she says that a little lidocaine jelly applied to the perineum three or four minutes before sex can ease discomfort. "Use until you're comfortable with vaginal estrogen."

Clearly you want to keep yourself clean, but there's no need to go further than water. Buy the wrong product for your vagina or vulva and you may cause more problems than you solve. A 2018 study by the University of Guelph in Canada found that ninety-five percent of women use products such as wipes, sprays, and creams at some point in their lives. But these seemed to come at some risk; those using gel sanitizers were eight times more likely to have a yeast infection and almost twenty times more likely to have a bacterial infection. Feminine washes or gels also increased the possibility of bacterial infection and urinary tract infections.

"Steaming is a terrible idea," adds Dr. Minkin. This was a huge trend a few years ago. "There were reports of second-degree burns to vaginas. Some celebrities were big proponents, but don't do it." To be honest, it's not just the thought that makes me flinch, but the sheer effort involved!

Buzzing Off

How is it not common knowledge that regular orgasms are more than just a fun pursuit? For a start, they can help with poor sleep—releasing a hormone called prolactin, which makes you feel relaxed. Sex helps with moodiness by both releasing oxytocin, a happy hormone, and reducing the stress hormone cortisol, as well as providing a handy inner workout.

Vibrators are not just a racy add-on to youthful sex, but another extremely valuable bedside drawer companion for middle-aged women. I have one friend who keeps her "Bullet"—a lovely little lipstick-shaped vibrator—in her handbag, in case the opportunity arises for a quickie in the loo during the workday. Is it a coincidence that she has never struggled with her sex life and she's now sixty-two? I think not.

You wouldn't think that our menopausal years would necessarily go hand in hand with experimental eroticism, but isn't that just another example of how we've been blindfolded by centuries of prejudice? If penetration is painful, then work around it. I don't think I need to explain in too much detail, but I do like the word "outercourse," which is nice and descriptive. In my early fifties, I spent six months compiling an anthology of erotica called *Desire*, and I can assure you my purpose was in equal measure selfish and magnanimous. It was also a glorious and sensual reawakening, during which time it was hard to entice me away from my "research."

I've heard single friends joking about their "virginity growing back" after a few months of no sex. In some ways, there's truth here in that the more you "use" your vagina, whether it's through sex or vibrators, the better.

"For those who haven't had sex for a long time, dilators can be very useful, and I'd encourage women to use them regularly," says Dr. Minkin. "Dilators are especially useful for cancer survivors; radiotherapy around the pelvic area can cause stenosis and scarring of the vagina, and I'd encourage women to speak to the radiotherapist about vaginal dilators, which help to keep it open, along with vaginal estrogen."

You certainly don't have to have a partner. Female masturbation is one of those taboo subjects, historically seen as either repulsive, dangerous to our delicate psyches (and, in Victorian times, could mean you got popped in an asylum if you were unlucky), or the stuff of male fantasy or porn films (often the same thing).

Intimate subjects are not easy to speak about, but thanks to public figures opening up it's becoming a more acceptable subject. "Addressing the taboo subject of vaginal dryness came about really slowly, and it was the thing I was most nervous about, thinking, 'Oh God, is that just a bit too icky?'" says actor and activist Naomi Watts. "But as I researched it, I learned that it's one of the most common symptoms and can lead to a lot of other issues, like the breakdown of a relationship because you're too scared to have sex; it's painful, but you don't feel brave enough to speak about it with your partner. Yet a simple solution—a squirt from a bottle of lube—can solve so much and not make you fear it so intensely. It's important to normalize all these once uncomfortable conversations. More lube for everyone I say!"

Naomi not only talks the talk but also walks the walk. Included in her pioneering Stripes line for women in midlife is a gel-based moisturizer, Vag of Honor, and Oh My Glide, a "play oil," both in beautiful, curved bottles that are nice enough to sit on your bedside table rather than shoved in its dark recesses! Naomi is not just tackling the overlooked aspects of women's health, but dispelling shame around it at the same time.

The benefits of masturbation are much the same as those achieved during sex. In fact, and I was delighted to read this in an article, though it seems an extrapolation too far, lower stress hormones mean you're less likely to stress eat, and therefore masturbation will help keep you thin. I'm not convinced by this, but I like the slightly convoluted logic. Are wankers less prone to gain weight? Nobody has yet done a definitive study on the subject, though there's a surprising amount of speculation, and sex *does* burn calories, though apparently only sixty-nine per session for women (such a marvelously appropriate number!).

All for the Pelvic Floor

The pelvic floor is the group of muscles in your pelvis that stretches across from pubic bone to backbone and supports the bladder, bowel, and uterus—all of which sit above it. Just like any other muscle group, the pelvic floor sags with age, and if it's out of shape, this can lead to leaking urine, as well as pelvic organ prolapse, where the bowel, uterus, bladder, or top of the vagina start to bulge downwards and can even protrude from the vagina. Constantly going to the bathroom at night is also associated with lack of pelvic-floor tone and lack of estrogen.

Women patients are very reluctant to introduce this topic, but, says Dr. Minkin, they are very grateful if you bring it up. "Urine leakage isn't glam or exciting, but very common in women as we age." There are two main problems, she explains. "Urge incontinence is where you have an overactive bladder; you need to go frequently and can't hold it in but—ironically—often can't empty the bladder." Think about when you have a bag of groceries and are desperately trying to unlock the door to get to the loo! "The other kind is stress incontinence, where you leak when you cough or sneeze." You can, incidentally, have both. Another problem is getting up every couple of hours at night to pee, particularly irritating if you are already struggling with insomnia. The trend for drinking massive amounts of water might be at fault in this last. "Some patients drink lots of water in the evening, which isn't a great idea. Start at noon, not eight p.m."

Women ideally need to learn about the pelvic floor long before menopause. "A good time to do pelvic-floor exercises is in your car when you stop at a stop sign," says Dr. Minkin. "Another patient told me that she does them when she puts gas in her car—one for every click. Every tank of gas I've put in since, I've done that." Basically, she says, squeeze the vaginal muscles as tightly as you can, elevating the pelvic floor to close the neck of the bladder. Try in the bathroom mid-pee to get an idea of what you're doing, but don't do them whilst peeing as it can lead to the bladder not emptying properly. "We used to think that Kegels only helped with stress incontinence, but they actually help with urge incontinence, too." Ideally do three sets of ten every day and try to hold for ten seconds.

Prolapse, where pelvic organs slip downwards and bulge into the vagina, can also cause leaking (as well as discomfort or pain). Data suggests that up to fifty percent of women will develop pelvic organ prolapse over their lifetime. "One of the things you can do is use pessaries," says Dr. Minkin. "There are all sorts—one looks like a giant contraceptive diaphragm, another like a flying saucer with the stem coming out. You need to figure out which works for you—it's rather like fitting shoes. They are inserted into the vagina and can be left for extended periods of time. Some women just use them if they're going to the gym or hiking." Most women can insert them by themselves, and you can have intercourse. "Some people—perhaps if they have severe arthritis—can't manage on their own, so they come to see me every three months." She says that she has many happy pessary patients. "There are surgical options, but most women prefer to try pessaries first."

You do not need to, nor should you, put up with incontinence. It's not simply an added ignominy of your later years. Address it right now or it *will* get worse. Too many of us see a little bit of leaking as our load to bear and behave as though it's not a big problem. But then you may stop exercising and having sex. As we get older and more frail, it becomes even more of an issue.

The problem is that women are used to dealing with pads and mess. We are sanguine about bodily fluids. But, left to its own devices, a sagging pelvic floor isn't going to resolve itself. Nothing, as those of us with muffin tops are aware, will tone itself. We joke about not being able to go on trampolines after a certain age, but there's no reason why most of us can't, if we work toward good inner muscle strength.

As muscles, including those of the pelvic floor, become weaker around menopause, there's no time to waste. I assume that you are doing those vital exercises right now—it's a reflex, like seeing somebody else yawn. "Squeeze the Day" was the inspirational slogan of a recently sponsored women's health campaign I took part in and it's now definitely my motto.

Most women have a favorite place to do a pelvic-floor workout. For example, I spend a great deal of time on a train en route to London from the West Country where I live, and I don't mind admitting it's an ideal moment for a few internal press ups. There are any number of apps that help you to remember and count them up on a daily basis, but I just do a few every time I remember or want to feel risqué in public!

"I've taken up reading steamy novels"

CARLA HALL, SIXTIES, CHEF, AUTHOR, TELEVISION HOST, WASHINGTON D.C.

I think that sex and relationships can get better as we age. We're more confident. I look up sometimes and I'm like, wow, I'm in my sixties. I know stuff. Admittedly I'd like to have more confidence in my sexual life. My husband and I have a really great relationship where we can talk about things, but I've spent so much time not saying "Hey, I want this or that" that I don't exercise that muscle. The biggest difference in perimenopause was my sex drive. I had a low libido anyway, and I was like "Oh my gosh, it's just gone!" It was really important for my husband and me to meld, so that was a huge part of the MHT decision. You need to keep your vagina working. The atrophy is real. I don't have vaginal dryness, which is great, and I think part of it is starting the hormones early.

Women need to be helped to understand their vaginas. This is where communication is so important. You hear a lot about penises, and if you aren't looking after the vagina, where the penises go, well, that's only half the equation. And certain terms are blocked on social media, which is where you can get a great deal of information, but anything about the female body, like vaginal dryness, you have to put a star to get it through the block!

One of the things I have owned is masturbation. I think, as an older woman, talking about it is important because it isn't discussed enough. I wasn't Catholic but I went to Catholic schools from kindergarten to ninth grade, so the shame around sex is real—and I grew up in the South, which doubles down on the shame. So part of my confidence in my relationship with myself is because I can masturbate. That comes from talking to my girlfriends and realizing how I'd slowed my sexual growth. I never listened to or read a romantic novel—give me a thriller or a Nancy Drew. But in this season that I'm in I decided to read and listen to audiobooks of steamy novels and it is so great! I'm talking to my friends and they're like "Girl, where have you been?" I feel like I'm just growing up.

"I had four years of agony"

LIZZIE, FIFTY-FOUR, TEACHER, NEW JERSEY

Over the years I've had lots of UTIs and I started getting them almost back-to-back about four years ago. It's no exaggeration to say that it plagues your life; feeling unwell, agonizing pain when peeing, and going to urgent care or to the doctor to get antibiotics the entire time. Sex was excruciating and I dreaded my husband suggesting it. My primary care doctor was no use, and just kept handing out antibiotics. Eventually I went to see a specialist who found vaginal atrophy. When she examined me, she said that, as I'd aged, my bladder, uterus, and vagina had been fighting for space, scrunched up and dry. She gave me estrogen cream to use at the entrance to the vagina. Since I started on that, I've not had a UTI, but it costs $100 per small tube. I feel resentful about the amount of time I spent in pain—I was naive not to have seen a specialist sooner, rather than assume my primary care doctor would know what was going on.

"Menopause has brought us closer together"

ANNA, FIFTY-EIGHT, ADVERTISING BUSINESS OWNER AND CCO, NEW YORK

Here's a positive. I think that my partner and I have become even closer during this process. It increased our communication level. A lot of women internalize and men don't understand what's happening. But articulating what was going on brought us closer. So with hot flashes, we started making fun of them. We used humor to elevate any tensions, because my hot flashes could burn a house down.

With vaginal dryness—which did occur—through communication we were like, well, sex is a multifaceted thing, and we worked around it. I think that his open-mindedness created this lovely bond in a way. It actually made our sex life stronger, because after many years together we started exploring!

CHAPTER ELEVEN

Hormonious Relationships

I have a dream but it begins as a nightmare. I start to experience a hot flash. My entire body is burning up in the fiery pits of hell (feels like). My partner is watching sympathetically. "Hot flash?" he asks, nicely, but not patronizingly, or annoyingly, thus balancing like a world-class trapeze artist on a gossamer-thin tightrope made from slender strands of optimism. "Shall I open a window and fetch you a glass of water?" "Thank you, darling," I say. "You understand me so well." We smile lovingly at each other and empty the dishwasher together. As I said, it's a dream!

Menopause isn't just about women. It affects everyone in your vicinity: partners, husbands, wives, children, and friends. This last group is—I feel—more likely to represent a pile of soft cushions for your emotions than target practice for sharp flashes of irritation. Originally, this chapter was going to be about partners, but actually menopause support takes a "village," so it's important to acknowledge and explore how all relationships might be impacted.

You don't need me to tell you that our moods affect those around us. During the years of menopause, elevated emotions, often negative or raging, might push us and those around us to the limits of endurance. It should be no surprise that women are more likely to take extreme action in midlife when it comes to relationships, whether in terms of divorce, abandoning long-term partnerships, or embarking on same-sex relationships for the first time.

Clearly, there's going to be a certain amount of misunderstanding between men and women because it's very hard to understand someone else's biology. But, speaking to lesbian couples, where both partners might be going through menopause at the same time, the unique experience of every woman means that there are obstacles to their mutual understanding, too.

If you have teenagers, who are by definition selfish and self-centered—this is science, by the way, not just weary observation—they may be bemused, loathe you a little more, or possibly even be curious about your mood swings. Sadly, it's unlikely they'll recognize their own pubescent ups and downs and sympathize. They'll definitely only be interested if it impacts them—whether it's taking advantage of your desperation for some peace or responding to ill-humor by hiding in their bedrooms until you've left the building. In all of these scenarios, when it comes to our relationships, I think menopause is ideally a time to breathe deeply before you utter a syllable, aim to educate, and look for those who might empathize. The greatest hurdle to wider understanding of what we're going through is often our reluctance to articulate it and ask for help and, even more fundamental, our ignorance of what's happening in our own bodies.

We'll start with men, whether they are husbands, partners, or boyfriends, because I am a heterosexual woman. It seems to me that not only are many men in near total ignorance of menopause, but that this state of affairs can be damaging to our relationships.

Why on earth shouldn't men know what's happening to women's bodies? If they experienced menopause, we'd definitely know about it! So, shouldn't they also be informed that one reason why their partner might be short-tempered or tired (or finding them sexually resistible) is because their hormones are going up and down like pistons? This is emphatically not so they can attribute any displays of exasperation to menopause, as has historically happened with this and PMS. Nothing is more guaranteed to infuriate than being patronized.

Some men still have a very bad habit of using the vagaries of women's biology as excuses for their own behavior. ("She's bad-tempered so I'm going to the pub.") Nevertheless, might it be worth recognizing that part of the eye-rolling, sniggering, and insensitivity on their part may disguise ignorance, concern, and slight trepidation about what is really happening to the woman they love?

Since women aren't exactly pouncing on the first signs of menopause as though it's the new Bond film, and our education is often as sparse as my knowledge of quantum physics, how on earth are men supposed to know what's happening?

I know that my husband is, on the whole, indifferent to the fluctuations of my hormones, unless they directly affect him. I have asked him how he found me during menopause, but unfortunately his answer was unprintable. For context, bear in mind that I believe I sailed through both my pregnancies joyously, one of the lucky minority for whom everything about gestation was a pleasure. Yet my husband describes me during those eighteen pregnant months as being unhinged, impossible to reason with, and in the grip of dark and malevolent forces. Imagine then how he'd outline a sleep-starved, terminally anxious, frequently bad-tempered, and entirely absentminded manifestation of me, without the promise of a new addition to the family at the end?

As I say, his response was unrepeatable.

Someone less generous in nature might argue that men's "midlife crises," with far less biological excuse, have been tolerated and even sympathized with throughout history. Imagine if they had a real physical reason to be distressed, and not just a burning desire to take up extreme sports, wear unseemly lycra outfits, and enlarge their automobile horsepower to prove they've still "got it"!

In a 2020 survey of fifteen hundred menopausal women and five hundred male partners, seventy-seven percent of the men said they'd noticed a change in their partner's moods, and fifty percent that their partner had gone off intimacy. A further forty percent noticed that their partner was always tired. Rather than being congratulated on their sensitivity and perceptiveness, these men often felt shut out. It also found that thirty-five percent of women only feel they can discuss menopause occasionally, rarely, or never. I'm surprised it's that many. I only asked my husband because of this book and his response guarantees I won't be asking again!

Interestingly, in 2019, the aptly named MATE (men's perception and attitudes toward menopause) survey found that men "are aware of their partner's menopausal transition," and concluded that they "could greatly benefit from additional training and/or resources."

Simply understanding what's happening can be a huge relief to us, so expanding that illumination to those in our immediate vicinity is ideal.

"My husband and I were at a conference in October 2023 where I was talking about menopause," says OB/GYN and midlife health expert Dr.

Taniqua Miller. "This was the first time I'd had a co-ed audience, and they were pretty much all in heterosexual marriages. And it was interesting because the men were asking all the questions in the wider group, and not just, 'What *is* this?' but really thoughtful ones, like 'How can I support my partner in this?' What I took away from this is that most partners want to understand what's happening and to support you, and they are really receptive to explanation."

Clearly, not every relationship is conducive to chatting about hormones, and this can be a personal or cultural consideration.

We asked a few men to speak to us about their feelings. Their responses were fascinating, but the overriding impression is one of vague misunderstanding. This simply confirms my suspicions that the best thing we can do is talk about menopause to our loved ones.

"Everything dries up"

JAMIE, FIFTY-TWO, INTERNATIONAL RELATIONS, SAN FRANCISCO

Yikes. Well, I don't know a huge amount about menopause—I've never been formally told about it, not even at school. My dad's an OB/GYN so it used to come up at the kitchen table every now and again. I remember my mom talking about it, though not her having strange moods or anything.

I think it's when the eggs stop being produced by the ovaries and everything—without being crass—dries up, and I think it happens in your late forties or early fifties, but I don't know how long the process takes. I've talked to my wife about it a little bit, mainly from a potential symptoms perspective, as in, "Could this be menopause?"

I'm hearing more and more about menopause lately, because my wife's friends are hitting that age. We went out on Saturday night and it came up in conversation. We're all a very close-knit group and the women are happy to talk about it in front of the men. Even so, there's lots of eye-rolling and "men are useless"—I think we're more tolerated than told about it!

"Is menopause responsible for midlife divorce?"

DAN, SIXTY-TWO, SALES DIRECTOR, NEW YORK

I read the *Wall Street Journal* and menopause is the kind of subject they'll cover. So, put it this way, I'm aware that it happens, and I directly see some of the effects on my wife. Sometimes she'll say that she's really hot, and she mentions hot flashes, and part of me thinks that's probably a side effect of menopause. We don't sit around and talk about it, but if she brings it up, I'm sympathetic.

I think it's fair to point out that you don't ask a woman if she's about to get her period. In the same way, you wouldn't suggest that a bad mood was menopause. You might be aware that something is going on, but you don't want to poke the bear. It's not worth the effort of the fight. There's probably a need for public education for men when it comes to the subject. A frightening amount of couples in their fifties and sixties split when kids go to college. Is menopause a part of that?

Midlife Split

Although it's obviously not possible for everyone, having experienced a parental breakup myself, I'm all for seeking balance in our existing relationships if we can. That said, "diamond divorce" and "silver splitters," where older couples separate, are clearly a "thing." Judging by the many letters I've received during my tenancy as an advice columnist for a national newspaper, women seem to feel a strong compulsion to embark on new challenges around menopause. Ending a long-term relationship rates quite highly among them. Interestingly, whatever age you are when you decide to call it a day, it's far more likely to be the woman behind the decision to divorce. Is it just me who finds that surprising? Popular mythology so often endorses the cliché of men finding younger models, but it's more likely to be females deciding that we're better off actually out of a marriage. In 2017, an analysis of over two thousand adults in a heterosexual marriage, "Who Wants

The Break Up?," confirmed that almost seventy percent of divorces were initiated by women. "Wives report lower relationship quality than husbands, while men and women in non-marital relationships report more similar relationship quality," said the author, Michael J. Rosenfeld, professor of sociology at Stanford University. Research also suggests that divorced women are happier afterward, even though financially they are likely to be worse off. Rather sweetly, marriage hasn't lost its charm. In 2022 there were 2,065,905 marriages across the forty-five US states that report this statistic, and 673,989 divorces and annulments. Interestingly, men are far more likely to remarry than women; 32 per 1,000 previously married men compared to 17.2 remarriages for women in 2021, which doesn't sound like much, but translates to over a million going down the aisle again. I salute them all, but must warn that second and third marriages are statistically more likely to fail.

Professor Rosenfeld found that there wasn't the same disparity between the sexes breaking up when in non-marital relationships. Same sex marriages have been legal across the States since 2015, and divorce rates tend to be slightly lower than those of heterosexual couples.

Now, clearly, I don't want to suggest that peri/menopause are responsible for the heterosexual divorce rate, but there's no question that "gray divorce"—that is, divorce among those over fifty—is on the rise. The combination of symptoms that can make you question your sanity with a delicious new devil-may-care attitude and sense of liberation from procreative and nurturing expectations are seemingly a compelling cocktail when it comes to our desire to change things up.

Some of the explanation for this may well be down to our maintaining traditional roles within marriage. "Feminist literature on marriage argues that heterosexual marriage is not only gendered, but fundamentally asymmetric and inegalitarian as well," said Professor Rosenfeld. He quoted Jessie Bernard's famous words (American sociologist 1903–1996): " 'There are two marriages, then, in every marital union, his and hers. And his . . . is better than hers.' Even between the most enlightened of couples this is likely to be the case."

Despite over a century of "leveling up" the sexes, this is proving a difficult dynamic to shift. When I think about my husband, certainly a hardworking and much-loved family man and nowadays primary cook, he is not the one doing the shopping lists, arranging pickups, scooping up the socks and damp towels from the bathroom floor, and putting the school events into our family calendar at the end of a hard day at the office. Yet we both work full-time.

I have also come across any number of postmenopausal women who are frustrated that their partners are happy to take the increasingly slow road to peaceful retirement, while they feel free at last, and want to travel the world, literally and metaphorically. And indeed, for many husbands, the absence of a "nurturing" partner comes as quite a shock! "I don't think of this time as a crisis, but as an awakening," says Dr. Miller. But for middle-aged men hoping to ease into their hobbies, renewed ambition can be disconcerting.

I've no desire to throw myself on the mercies of the single silver-haired foxes of the English countryside, where I live, or indeed anywhere beyond my own backyard, but I'd be lying if I didn't admit to recognizing the appeal in choosing to be with someone who does have an interest in your dirty laundry—no pun intended.

If a marriage or relationship is loveless, toxic, and irreparable, it's often better that it comes to a dignified end, especially for the sake of children. But with my advice columnist hat on, I'd suggest doing everything possible to avoid this outcome. Divorce is usually expensive and extremely stressful. For midlife women influenced by mood swings, inexplicable rage, and all the other emotional side effects of perimenopause, thinking that their subliminal woes will be solved by a partner reboot, it would be irresponsible not to remind you that the grass is rarely greener. So don't let a passing period of hormonal turbulence dictate actions that you may live to regret. Divorce should be a final act, taking place only when all other possibilities have been exhausted: couples' counseling, mediation, and a final holiday together!

That last is no joke; I know a couple who lived together in name only for six years for the sake of their kids, and then, on a road trip to visit mutual friends in Italy, rediscovered their mojo. I find it utterly heartwarming when I see them in the local park, walking hand in hand, looking like teenagers in love. So, never say never, especially if there's a vacation involved!

On the flip side, I know plenty of supersmart New Yorkers who got itchy feet, ditched their husbands, and lost the house in the Hamptons and all their friends in one swoop, though, clearly, these are first-world problems and not the average experience. And if "friends" abandon you that quickly they're not worth treasuring anyway! Despite self-help-style encouragement to "find yourself," you won't automatically skip off into a land populated entirely by handsome and solvent fifty-year-olds without a trail of toxicity and three truckloads of battered emotional baggage behind them.

This is not to say that if you're unhappy in a relationship you should grit your teeth and dig in. Plenty of women have found contentment and new partners after divorce, and good luck to them. But sexism in the post-menopausal years is never more evident than in the sphere of dating. A dear friend in her fifties, recently divorced, dipped her toe into the world of online dating. "All the women were in their forties and fifties and incredibly glamorous. 'Running a multinational company and looking for Mr. Right' was the vibe," she tells me. "The men, on the other hand, were mostly balding, over sixty, and looked like the cat had got the cream. Positives tended to be along the lines of 'has own teeth.'"

This is just an example, and there are plenty of dating agencies with more balance, and swathes of exciting-looking eligible bachelors, but, even so, single girlfriends in their fifties tell me that it's not an even playing field out there, and at times it's a desert. And unless your personal oasis is a man a good decade older, who feels that he's lowered his expectations, then true love isn't necessarily a given. As for the trend in dating far younger men . . . If it's for you, then go forth. Personally, I'd struggle displaying my wrinkly carcass to someone new (and I'm fairly sure that this might be a mutual feeling), but I can't help admiring those who follow their hearts, or whatever else is doing the instructing in that instance.

An example is film star and author Joan Collins, whose most enduring and by all accounts happy marriage has been to Percy Gibson, a man thirty-two years her junior. On being asked about the age difference, she famously quipped, "If he dies, he dies."

New relationships soon start to resemble old ones, and all too often the real emotional renovations required are internal rather than external. Reinvention can be a path to personal happiness. Along with the huge challenges for couples navigating their middle years, there are equally large benefits for those who successfully do so. To those who separate and manage to companionably negotiate their way through their post-divorce years, I applaud you. Here's to a happy and companionable old age, whatever way you manage to achieve it!

Think of the Children

As we lose the hormones that exist to help us reproduce, oxytocin, the hormone that helps us bond with our children and increases when we fall in love, also goes down. Do we become less cuddly and more driven? Perhaps more "masculine" or focused in our outlook? We have spoken to women who say that obviously they still love their offspring, but in a more detached fashion, not that blind adoration you have for tiny babies or hapless toddlers.

Just remember that children are incredibly sensitive to mood change, and they need to understand what's happening as well. Find the common ground, says Dr. Miller. "If someone is going through the menopausal transition and has increased irritability and anxiety, you might also have a teenager going through their own hormonal transition, with increased irritability and anxiety at the same time. It's great for folks to be on the same page." She says that recognizing that it's a similar process, having open lines of communication, and giving each other some grace will be hugely beneficial.

You need to look after yourself, she reminds us. "There can be a lot of disembodiment if you're in the throes of menopause. I have one patient who described it as though she was outside of herself and looking down at herself. I think of psychologist Abraham Maslow's hierarchy of needs. If your psychological and physical needs aren't being met—basic levels of survival like sleep, eating well, exercising, and having safety in relationships, how can you pour love and belonging into your children?"

Or, she says think of yourself as being a vessel that you fill up every morning. "Sometimes it's half full, but as you're walking and being pulled in all directions, there's water pouring out. I think sometimes when people are going through the menopausal transition and have all these things happening to them, they don't have an opportunity to go back to the well and fill up. So you're depleted, and there's nothing left to pour out."

"If you are feeling shame about irritability and maybe avoiding your children, slow down and ask yourself: What do I need right now? Then you can start pouring back into the vessel."

I know that, in my late forties, pre-MHT, when my two were still very young, and therefore hopefully didn't notice as much, I was probably snappier than I should have been, because of lack of sleep, anxiety, and stress. I've already mentioned that my daughter thinks I threw a book at her during my perimenopausal years, and I stand by the fact that I think it's a false memory on her part! Joking aside, there is a platitude that a happy mother means happy children, which I take to mean that women should do as much as they can to be happy (while enormously checking my own privilege and understanding that there are many things outside our control). "You are human, you aren't perfect," says Dr. Miller. "Explain to them when you have those moments where you feel really irritable. Of course, with teenagers, this isn't always going to be menopausal madness, but justified annoyance at lateness or untidiness. Tell them!"

The goal, as with husbands and partners, is to give an explanation so that those around you realize that it's not their fault. That said, when you're in the midst of a storm, you don't necessarily realize you are the one causing waves.

Talk to the Teens

I asked parenting expert Tanith Carey, author of *What's My Teenager Thinking?*, why it's so hard to talk to our teens about any discomforts. "Because we find menopause a difficult, intimate, and sensitive topic, we often assume it's not a 'need-to-know' for teens," she says. "We tend to hope that their biology syllabus will cover it. Even if it does come up, it will still seem very one-dimensional to them. Kids need to understand it's an actual thing that is happening to you and other women your age." The median age to have a baby in the US is thirty, which means that many women are going through the upheavals of perimenopause at the same time their children hit puberty. "On top of that, research shows the task of setting limits for teens already falls more to mothers than fathers—and teens tend to be more antagonistic toward female parents."

So, all in all, the barrage of criticism, often mixed with contempt, which is part of the normal process of separation for teens from their parents, becomes harder to bear. This can also make this period of parenting feel particularly tough, says Carey. "It is an age when we may already be feeling less confident, and as though we're losing our bloom, while watching our daughters blossom—so we are often bearing the brunt of our children's adolescence at a very vulnerable time in our lives."

The thought of their mother having periods may sound "gross" to your teen, perhaps even grosser when she stops, not to mention the fact that, at their age, empathy doesn't come naturally. "Developmentally they have to be incredibly self-centered. It's a vital step toward cutting loose on their own and becoming independent."

"Teens also like to think they are the only people in the house going through anything difficult. So their first instinct, when they hear that you may be more tired or are having a tough time, is less likely to be 'I can see she needs some rest,' and more likely to be 'What about me?!'" Teens are still developing their "theory of mind"—the ability to imagine what life feels like for other people—while, as I've described already in our menopause years, we're blissfully shedding ours. The fact that menopause feels a long way off to a teenager means they are unlikely to be particularly curious or want to hear about it.

Rather than feeling frustrated that they're being so selfish, understand that it's par for the course, says Carey. "Be matter-of-fact: rather than being dramatic about menopause, refer to it naturally in daily conversation rather than a sit-down-facts-of-life-heart-to-heart. So, if your daughter is talking about her own period starting that month, mention perhaps that you haven't had one for a while (and what a relief that is!). With boys, use some humor to say you need to remove some facial hair, too, because you are also sprouting more of it as you furiously rub on the testosterone that your body is discarding! Though your teen may not appreciate your candor at first, adopt a tone of 'we are all in this together,' and use it to open conversations about life stages more generally and ask them questions about what they're going through."

Friends Are for Life, Not Just for Fun

Then there is friendship. Whether you choose to go it alone in later life and enjoy the benefits of independence, renewed confidence, and new horizons, or work at reforming and reinvigorating your current relationship, there are those who will still be there for you through thick and thin. My girlfriends have been the life raft that's kept me afloat for nearly four decades now, and while they were fun and frivolous and perfect playmates in my twenties, as the years progress, they have become so much more important than that. I found a study looking at women in recovery, and it concluded that the stronger women's friendships, the higher their self-esteem, hope, and social support, which came as no surprise to me.

I used to rent a country house with a lesbian couple, where I spent the majority of my singleton thirties, and where some of my happiest memories were made. At the time we would joke that we were going to join together to buy a house in Tuscany, to which we would retire in our dotage. It would be staffed by gloriously attractive nurses of both sexes, and we'd idle away our twilight years behaving outrageously, drinking martinis at breakfast, and possibly nurturing addictions to the illegal drugs we'd avoided until then, or at least taking copious quantities of the ones we could get prescribed. Sharing our booty of sleeping pills, antidepressants, and whatever else we could get our debauched paws on, could be one of our daily activities, along with cheating at cards. This hasn't yet come to pass, but I still think, as a dream, it's an excellent one. In reality, a close-knit community of people around you, who know you, accept your faults, celebrate your virtues, and can prop you up when knockout blows come along, is key to a healthy, happy existence from midlife and beyond. So, as much as we expect our romantic partners and children to understand what's going on during menopause, it's also important to inform our friends, and perhaps by doing so spread the weight of our needs. There is no better way of easing the pressure than airing and sharing your woes, and I've been amazed these last ten years to find so many women initially shy to confide, and then unstoppable when it comes to detailing the ups and downs, trials and tribulations of the hormonally unbalanced years.

"A positive of this time of life is being surrounded by the women you've had years and years of history with," agrees Naomi Watts. "I've just had a wonderful gathering of friends where we allowed ourselves to be goofy: it was stupid, base, low-level humor. But what was really in the room was an unbelievable amount of love. It's incredibly emotional. Nothing is more anchoring than those women that you've grown up with and sharing things, whether it's ups or downs, lots of important stories that have changed us. We've stayed together over the years, and I'm proud of being able to hold on to those friendships."

As seen in movies from *Thelma and Louise* to *Beaches*, *Bridesmaids*, and *Booksmart*, the pleasure older women find in companionship is matched only by the intensity of teenage buddies who tell each other everything. I'd say it's even more satisfying when you're older, because you know how precious friendships are. Alice and I toyed with the idea of calling this book "Help! I'm Hormonally Unbalanced." For proof that friendships are imperative, look no further than what you are reading: an enterprise dreamed up in a running group started among some middle-aged school mums. Our weekly outings, where we generally talk faster than we run, have been a rallying lifeline for each one of us at various times over the last seven years: through divorce, mental illness, issues with children, death, and health scares. If you do decide that, when it comes to your romantic relationship, it's out with the old, make sure that, when it comes to friendships, you treasure longevity.

"The menopause 'filter' warped everything"

SUSIE, SIXTY, LEARNING AND DEVELOPMENT
PROFESSIONAL, DELAWARE

For me, menopause was defined by that white-hot rage that flares up out of nowhere, which meant I had an overexaggerated and disproportionate response to innocuous questions. So, for example, my husband might ask, "Are you going into the office today?" A fair question you'd think. But through the filter of having hot flashes, not having any sleep or any sex and feeling utterly unattractive as well as fuzzy-headed, I would process it as "Your job is incidental, you don't earn as much as I do, you might as well stay at home painting your nails and do you even contribute to society?" So I would defend my existence, and he would retreat, cowed, muttering, "I only *asked*."

This lasted a decade, but in the last two years it's calmed down. I realize that I'm responding normally to situations and then realize it's probably because I'm out of it now and more chill about things.

"We have to talk to our partners"

LINDSAY MABRY, FORTY-EIGHT, ACTOR, TEXAS

My mother doesn't talk about anything. It's a generational thing, and I think it was ingrained in them not to say anything negative. I remember saying to my grandmother that my doctor thought I might have postnatal depression. And she said, "Oh well, that didn't exist back in my time."

And yet I absolutely think it's helpful to speak to family and to our partners. I mentioned menopause to my husband; I said, you're going to have to understand that my body is sort of attacking itself and doesn't feel so good. I can't help it some days, and I need you to support me. Men can't read our minds, and they need us to be more direct.

I speak with close friends, and I'm always grateful when they have the courage to speak about it as well—then you get the advice. I spoke to a friend about menopause this summer when we were down by the river with the kids. She said she gets this unexplained rage, and I said, me too. I have no reason for the rage. I love my life and my family, but it's just what my body is doing at the moment.

CHAPTER TWELVE

Facing the Future

We hope by now you're feeling considerably better informed and less apprehensive about menopause, whatever age or stage you're at. Having put the myths in their place (mostly, the nineteenth century), sorted the MHT scaremongering, and slotted the myriad symptoms into some semblance of order, there's no reason not to step forth with a lighter heart and a better-stocked brain and bathroom cabinet or bedside drawer. But being better equipped to survive menopause is not enough. Who's up for a celebration?

In the award-winning show *Fleabag*, there is a blazing summary of menopause delivered by actor Kristin Scott Thomas. "It may be the best three minutes of television ever; any woman over forty-five, or under forty-five, should have it on a loop," said the *LA Times* in 2019. "Menopause," says Kristin, to an incredulous, martini-sipping Phoebe Waller-Bridge, ". . . is the most wonderful fucking thing in the world, and, yes, your entire pelvic floor crumbles and you get fucking hot, and no one cares, but then you're free, no longer a slave, no longer a machine with parts—you're just a person, in business . . . It is horrendous, but then it's magnificent . . . Something to look forward to."

And she's absolutely right. For some (hopefully now ready to take advantage of the support available), the journey won't always be pleasant, but emerging on the other side can be life-affirming and even cause for euphoria. We said at the beginning that, throughout history, there have been too few women's voices on the subject of menopause, and no wonder. For good reason most felt it far better to keep quiet and suffer than be reviled, locked up, or—even worse—"healed" with one of the life-threatening "cures" on offer.

The normalization of menopause is to be hugely celebrated. I, for one shouted an *Hallelujah* whilst watching the 2024 Super Bowl, where menopause drug Veozah took a sixty-second advertising slot alongside Uber Eats, Volkswagen, and Hellmann's. It was certainly a reminder of the burgeoning commercialization of menopause and the gleeful involvement of pharmaceutical companies; with every successful societal integration comes the pile on of businesses jumping on the bandwagon. To be targeting midlife women at such a celebrity-studded and high-profile event on a topic once deemed unmentionable shows just how far menopause has traveled in our collective psyche.

When women themselves have shared their feelings about getting older, they generally sound far less traumatized than "experts" down the centuries have declared we should be. In reality, plenty have faced the concept of their advancing years with cheery equanimity and enjoyed a perfectly happy and productive later life. It's just that the voices of (mostly) female doctors, sociologists, writers, and campaigners haven't been heard as loudly as the booming voices of doom. And now, as our place in society improves, equity seems a possibility and we're "allowed" to vote, have careers, and are generally in charge of our own destinies, it's often in the postmenopause years that we get to reap the benefits and come into our own.

Of course, there are discomforts, and there are the distraught case studies published by doctors, but the official depiction of desperate, lust-ridden, shriveled witches, burning with shame at being of no use to man nor beast has been hugely oversold.

Positive female voices about menopause may start out as murmurs, but, as the centuries pass, there is a gathering public roar of acknowledgment that our post-ovulation years don't constitute a sad and redundant phase. Instead, it's an era to be anticipated, freed from the shackles of our biological inheritance.

This has been pointed out by a few authors, who have taken the time to delve deep. It was acknowledged at various times in the dark days of the past that after the "madness" might come contented old age (and even a happy move toward being more like a man!), but women sometimes took it further. In *The Curse: A Cultural History of Menstruation*, American feminist and suffragette Eliza Farnham is referenced. She wrote about menopause in the 1860s, calling it "a time of 'secret joy,' of 'super-exaltation.'"

Then there's famed women's rights campaigner Marie Stopes, who opened the UK's first birth control clinic in 1921. In her book *The Change of Life*, published the same year, she says: "Judging by their exhortations most writers for climacteric women have very little knowledge of health and sanity and their exhortations are often extremely dangerous to women. So in bold print I am going to emphasise: **Do not anticipate any trouble at all at this time of life.**" Of course, we had only just been given the vote when she dared put her head above the parapet. I am naturally reeling with surprise. So . . . the men were exaggerating?

Anthropologist Margaret Mead referred to the power of "postmenopausal zest" in the 1950s, and in 1963, the psychologist Bernice Neugarten led a piece of research showing that many postmenopausal women felt better after menopause than they had in years, feeling generally calmer and happier.

In the last few years, there has been a veritable cacophony of positivity. We're finally celebrating this liberating time of life, when the world becomes our oyster, rather than our retirement home. Menopause, having come in from the cold, is now the hottest of topics. We hear public figures, from heavyweight politicians to celebrities, speaking about the subject at every available opportunity. Michelle Obama talked about her own hot flashes in a 2020 groundbreaking podcast conversation with OB/GYN Dr. Sharon Malone. "What a woman's body is taking her through is important information. It's an important thing to take up space in a society, because half of us are going through this but we're living like it's not happening."

When Michelle speaks, everybody listens. If she can chat about her hot flashes as though it's no more of an issue than the weather, then millions of us are nodding along in relief. "When women have the power to speak out without being discriminated against, it changes the dynamic immeasurably," says Dr. Malone. "We are not just going to be quiet and slink away, and I think that the more positive role models we have of women who are of a certain age and who are vibrant, beautiful, and still out there and being very much part of the work world and the political world, the better. We are shedding that cloak of invisibility that generations before us have had to shoulder."

The more it's publicly discussed, the more acceptable the conversation. In 2023, the magnificent Drew Barrymore memorably had her first ever hot flash whilst interviewing Jennifer Aniston and Adam Sandler on TV. In 2019, Oprah said of menopause, "I've discovered that this is your moment to reinvent yourself after years of focusing on the needs of everyone else." Actor Gillian Anderson wrote a book with her friend Jennifer Nadel called *We*—a manual for women seeking happiness, saying: "Perimenopause and menopause should be treated as the rites of passage that they are . . . If not celebrated, then at least accepted and acknowledged and honored." Gwyneth Paltrow, who has endured ridicule for her frank discussion of all aspects of women's experience, was positively pioneering in 2018 with her understatement: "Menopause gets a really bad rap and needs a bit of rebranding." Actor Tracee Ellis Ross has spoken about reaching perimenopause and being childless. "I can feel my body's ability to make a child draining out of me," she said. And of course, there's the magnificent Naomi Watts, whose words you've already heard in the foreword to this book.

The noisier the better, and the more the better, is what I say. We're owning this; following on from millennia of rigid-lipped reticence, or confidently proclaimed, but generally baseless, views from those who will never experience menopause.

In the process of making the 2018 BBC documentary, writing this book, and campaigning in the UK and now in the US, I've heard and read about hundreds, even thousands, of similar voices: politicians, chefs, store assistants, teachers, doctors, nurses, celebrities, those sharing information on Facebook groups and websites, and those writing books. All of them were equally content to communicate about this too-long-buried secret. If you laid all the women now speaking about menopause end to end, I'd say we'd wrap around the world, and what a great advantage that would be. A planet surrounded by mature, wise, and worldly women might be a better place for all of us.

Not only is it acceptable to talk openly and enthusiastically about menopause, but let's also point out the proven positives to later life.

Happier in Every Way

We are likely to be happier as we age. This is borne out by a great deal of scientific data, even though happiness is surely so subjective that it's near impossible to accurately define. In the US its pursuit is your constitutional right! According to a 2023 study involving over 460,000 participants from different countries and cultures, life satisfaction goes down from nine to sixteen, then increases a little until the age of seventy. After this point it's on the decrease, I'm afraid, until the age of ninety-six (or death, whichever comes first).

This phenomenon is explained in an analysis conducted by psychologist and academic Katherine Campbell at the University of Melbourne in Australia. This traced the happiness and health of a group of four hundred women, from their mid-forties to mid-fifties, for twenty years, and found that contentment grew along with the decades accrued.

"Women feel more in control of their lives and are still physically capable of enjoying their hobbies and traveling. They are often more financially stable and have less responsibility for children," she said. "They are free to enjoy the fruits of their hard work and are able to prioritize their own needs and wants."

Another 2017 Australian study, with four hundred women aged forty to sixty, also showed that postmenopausal women have a far more positive view of the transition than premenopausal. The authors pointed out that "Given the association between representations and bothersomeness of menopausal symptoms, clinicians should educate women about their expectations, and challenge their negative beliefs about menopause."

Incidentally, there are also plenty of studies into confidence, and, again, the older woman very much comes out on top. Our confidence increases—and so it should—with age and experience.

In 2019, Harvard Business Review reported research whereby data had been collected from more than four thousand women and three thousand men since 2016. Only around thirty percent of women aged twenty-five or younger said they felt confident, with around half of men saying the same. Remember that sheer insecurity of being twenty-five, an age for which I'd suggest the term "imposter syndrome" could have been coined?

We equalize by forty, but then, and this is the interesting bit, by the age of sixty, women tend to surpass men in confidence. Male confidence grows just eight and a half percentile points between the ages of twenty-five and sixty-plus, but female confidence increases by twenty-nine percentile points. It suggests that having navigated menopause, women are actually emboldened to face other challenges. There really is a lot to look forward to and, as the latter proves, it's not just hearsay.

Later Life Taking Flight

Although reality shows and social media might suggest otherwise, it is entirely possible to enjoy a full and successful career later in our life cycle, and I don't just mean Meryl Streep and Helen Mirren, who are always brought out and dusted off as older sex symbols and fine examples of how postmenopausal women can still work and, in Mirren's case, wear red bikinis.

Kamala Harris became the first woman to take such an elevated elected office when she became vice president of the United States in 2021, aged fifty-six, having previously been successful throughout her career as a lawyer, district attorney, and senator. Director Kathryn Bigelow hit the big time in 2008, aged fifty-seven, when she directed *The Hurt Locker*. Stylist Patricia Field was fifty-four when she met Sarah Jessica Parker and the pair were catapulted into award-winning fashion nirvana during the heady *Sex and the City* years of the late nineties. She's since been nominated for five Emmys. And Arianna Huffington founded the Huffington Post when she was in her fifties. Age isn't, and shouldn't be, an impediment to career goals and success.

"My mantra is 'Say yes. Adventure follows, then growth,'" says chef, author, and television host Carla Hall. "Own and take control of your life, even at the point when you feel you're over the hill. You're not—because you have all this wisdom. I think that my mantra helps me to accept change in my body."

I know from my own experience that, although my work goals may have changed, I'm far more industrious (and more health conscious) than I ever was; I prioritize differently. I love what I do, but I also relish being with my family. There isn't the same sense of FOMO if I don't go to someone's party or the latest must-attend event. My contemporaries share a deeply committed work ethic, but also the ability to separate work and play quite firmly. If you can't put your foot down about family time when you're over fifty, then when can you? And it doesn't mean I'm any less ambitious, driven, or focused.

Take Note of Money

Spend those pennies. The money we have managed to accrue over the years is vital to the economy. As lifespan and working life extends, your dollars have never been more valued. A look at the Federal Reserve's 2023 Survey of Consumer Finances shows that the wealthiest age band is sixty-five to seventy-four, with a median net worth of $409,000, and the second wealthiest is fifty-five to sixty-four at $364,500. This second group also has the highest median income—$91.9K. According to the AARP Longevity Economy Outlook reports, consumers aged fifty-plus contribute $8.3 trillion to the economy each year. As Forbes.com points out, women dominate consumer purchasing decisions—driving seventy to eighty percent of all decisions. Ignore us at your peril.

Who knew that our power extends to our disproportionate contribution to the economy! As the most powerful consumers—it's high time we started flexing that muscle.

Not only are we spending on leisure services and travel, but we're also the ones to watch when it comes to actively supporting employment and making money—and therefore holding up the economy. (It's at this point that I fervently hope younger women will read the book and understand that getting older and a bit more wrinkly doesn't diminish your importance.) The Longevity Economy® Outlook found that in 2018, people aged fifty and older supported 88.6 million jobs in the US, through jobs they hold or create, directly or indirectly. What's more, people aged fifty-plus contributed $745 billion worth of unpaid activities such as volunteering and caregiving across the country. In addition, people aged fifty-plus made $97 billion in charitable contributions in 2018. They spent—deep breath—$135 billion on educational services, including for their children and grandchildren, and contributed $4 billion to educational institutions across the United States. That hardly suggests that we're all sitting at home browsing catalogs and counting the quarters we've hidden under our stained mattresses. What a shame that business hasn't yet woken up to the power of the postmenopausal dollar!

We may be solvent and employed, but it will come as no surprise to discover that our power and wealth isn't being reflected in advertising or television. Only five to ten percent of marketing budgets target our age group, in spite of us representing more than half of consumer spending. Another literal example of older people being undervalued.

Women are also underrepresented across all forms of media. If you want your blood to boil, find one of those charts that shows how much dialogue women are given in top-billing films versus men.

In 2022, only ten percent of films featured a woman aged forty-five or older as the lead or co-lead, says research done by the University of Southern California's Inclusion Initiative. And the 2024 Gender in Advertising Report by CreativeX showed women in family settings nineteen percent of the time and only 3.4 percent of the time in leadership roles. Tedious, isn't it? Older women featured in fewer than two percent of advertisements, and when present they were twice as likely to be in domestic roles. Given the afore-mentioned spending power of this group, it appears that advertising needs to get with the program. I for one don't feel motivated to buy fashion and beauty products when they're advertised to me by girls a quarter of my age.

Changing Face of Beauty

Older women look fantastic when they're feeling buoyant and confident within themselves, but that doesn't lessen the joy of welcoming the innovation of menopause beauty products. Even a few years ago, face creams specifically for menopausal skin were virtually unheard of. Companies didn't want to mention the word let alone target those in its ravaging clutches! Who wants to make creams for shriveled has-beens? Happily, thanks to some forward-thinking pioneers, things have changed.

The beauty industry, which I must cynically point out does little product development purely from the goodness of its own heart, appears to be embracing menopause as a new cash bonanza. There are positive overtones of change in the very fact that there's active investigation into the needs of mature and menopausal skin, though some of the advertising leaves a lot to be desired. We don't all become born-again Victorian ladies in middle age, hankering after rose water and lavender bags! Still too much of the mature-woman packaging tends toward the pastel and the floral—a little too redolent of nineteenth-century doctors calming us down with smelling salts and a good paternal talking to! However, it's extremely heartening that menopausal makeup and skincare has become a booming business. At the forefront are pioneers such as Naomi Watts and the ever-inspiring Bobbi Brown. In many ways Brown is a perfect case study for the potential of the mature woman. Having sold her eponymous company, in her sixties she embarked on a whole new business dedicated to older skin called Jones Road. There's also Caire Beauty, Alloy, and Paula's Choice . . . the list goes on.

"Skin is one of the first things that really became a problem in my menopause journey," says Naomi Watts, who created her Stripes line specifically for menopausal women in 2022. "And my skin is so important, being on camera so often. I was forty-seven, and already having extreme symptoms. My skin was itching, inflamed, and irritated. So I changed my skincare routine first—switching to all sorts of gentle and clean ingredients. I started reading these labels, and the ingredients were all stripping and drying. It doesn't make sense for a woman who's going through this. I also went to the dermatologist a few times, and he sent me away with ointments that were soothing for a day or two. I started doing the deep dive and realized that it was all related. That's what led me to developing Stripes."

She says that she was surprised by the enthusiasm of investors. "I'll never forget the first meeting, where I had to do a cold pitch with people I'd never met before. I think there were at least two men on the call, and I was terrified about how it would be received. But I came in really well prepared. I knew that half the population is going to experience this at some point, and the fact that the secret had been held so tightly for so many generations made absolutely no sense. I pointed out that there's a hydration issue from scalp to vag (yes, I said vagina). I could see people's eyes light up, and they said yeah, we want to do this, before the meeting had even ended."

Such hallowed websites as Vogue.com are riddled with references to menopause beauty. One brilliant science-led feature about skincare for estrogen-drained skin on Oprah Daily had me desperately trying to source Alloy products from the States. "I am always pointing to women who are incredibly chic and have lines on their face," says editorial director of Oprah Daily, Pilar Guzmán. "Jane Fonda not dyeing her hair . . . Andie MacDowell going gray . . . now she's like 'fuck it.' I think the more people who do that and who look chic—it's redefining the aesthetic and the ideal of beauty at this age. And the more that we can represent those women in movies as being the ones to emulate, the better."

However, with such welcome new product development comes deep cynicism and concern that menopausal women are being exploited, with companies slamming the word on spurious products and vulnerable consumers snapping them up.

The global menomarket was estimated to be worth $17.8 billion in 2023 and is growing faster even than the list of potential symptoms. Meno-themed products include shakes, supplements, vaginal moisturizers, cooling mists, and shampoos. Some are magnificent, while some companies are clearly joyfully cashing in. We're not saying don't buy them—buy whatever you like, but read the small print. They might not be as innovative as they initially appear.

Excitingly, there is even a movement against the term "anti-aging." Some magazines are even recommending the use of the term "pro-aging"—which is about the acceptance that women would like to look the best they can, rather than twenty years younger. Even age-defying will do, in its slightly revolutionary suggestion. What with aging being an irrefutable fact of life, how wonderful if this were the start of a sea change in the perception of beauty. I'm not quite able to be at the forefront of this particular battle. I suspect I may still be clutching the peroxide bottle on my deathbed, but relaxing the fight against wrinkles would be very empowering! In one hundred years' time, perhaps our crow's feet will be perceived as coveted marks of maturity, as they are with those handsome rugged older men used for advertising expensive watches, rather than a failure of lifestyle, genetics, and personal maintenance when it comes to the female of the species.

Brighter Brains

Intelligence can also increase with age. You don't have to think of the post-menopausal years as being those where you constantly search your handbag for keys and your head for the right word (though I do more than my fair share of both). Research now tells us that there is no reason to assume that your mind is fading, even if you were unfortunate enough to suffer from (or still do) the brain fog that can descend with diminishing estrogen.

Neuroplasticity is basically the brain's ability to learn and adapt, and this continues throughout life. However, when we're older, we also have the benefit of what's called crystallized intelligence. This grows with age—it will peak around sixty or seventy and is the ability to combine knowledge and experience to approach new problems, hence the wisdom recognized by the grandmother hypothesis. This is also one of the many reasons why agism, especially in the workplace, is so misplaced.

What a relief to learn that, after decades of gorging on literature for my BBC book show, activities like reading tangibly increase intelligence, keeping the brain active and slowing the decline of age. Not only does reading improve your mind and maintain agility, but it is linked to longevity. A study of more than 3,500 people found that reading a book for thirty minutes a day adds a couple of years to your lifespan. It's also said that reading every day means that you are less likely to develop Alzheimer's. Happily, I love reading, and if it counts as brain training then all the better.

Epilogue

In summary, and with enormous satisfaction, I would like to confirm that the times really are changing and the rebrand of the transition is well on its way. We need to adapt, too, and stop scuttling around in shame, trying to hide the evidence that we're no longer available for procreative purposes. Evolution has designated us far more valuable than the sum of our eggs, and it's high time we embraced that accolade and stopped being apologetic for reaching our perceived sell-by date. The first step must be to take control, steer ourselves comfortably through, and finally celebrate this rewarding phase in our lives that leads only to further liberation. I am over the moon that so many more women are standing up to be counted as loud, proud, and menopausal, and thank goodness the conversation shows no sign of abating. I now believe that menopause might just have been the best thing to happen to me. So let's redefine it as a fresh start and the gateway to an exciting future about which we are delighted to proclaim.

Having been through menopause and emerged to find the sun still shining on the other side, I can assure you that it is not the inescapable black hole or end of the line train station I originally assumed. Quite the opposite in fact. Equipped with knowledge and the right tools, menopause can be an ultimately enriching passage, culminating in a more confident and happier life, despite the unavoidable aches and pains and irritating symptoms that mark this transitional phase.

I think I'm probably healthier, happier, and fitter than I've ever been, barring three months in my thirties when I fancied a man at the local gym and barely left the treadmill for fear of missing him.

Along with celebration, we need to start demanding change in the treatment, or should that be mistreatment, of so many women after centuries of misinformation and malpractice. I never want to hear another anecdote about a doctor's appointment that ends with the patient being told that the doctor doesn't agree with MHT and fobbing her off with a prescription for antidepressants.

If this book highlights anything, it should be the importance of education for all, consistency in ensuring the right information is produced, and availability of support for anyone who needs it.

This trio of knowledge might help bring an end to the sense of terror, embarrassment, and ignorance many of us feel at the onset of what's simply a midlife readjustment.

I like Omisade Burney-Scott's description of this time of life where the older woman is likened to the crone and goddess-based traditions. "The crone is the wise woman who has all the lived experiences and is associated with the dark side of the moon." We should all embrace our inner or (more likely the older we get) our outer crone.

Or there's the modern interpretation of traditional Chinese medicine which declares that our postmenopausal years should be viewed as a second spring, which Chinese medicine practitioner Katie Brindle tells me is a metaphor used extensively to describe this time. I won't belabor the point, as the imagery is pretty obvious: green shoots, fresh approaches, renewed vigor, and so on.

I even found a passage describing the process, which she says appears to derive from a translation of the *Yellow Emperor's Classic of Internal Medicine* (originally written around 2600 BC).

At seven times seven a woman's heavenly dew wanes;
the pulse of her Conception channel decreases.
The Qi that dwelt in the baby's palace moves upward into her heart,
and her wisdom is deepened.

It is a shame, of course, to lose one's heavenly dew, but the idea of becoming more powerful, knowledgeable, and with stacks of deep wisdom is one that I, and hopefully all of you, eagerly anticipate.

Understanding the historical culture that's led us down our current cul-de-sac of fear and ignorance is half the fight. Celebrating future freedom requires a further shift away from the status quo. Navigating your way across this occasionally choppy sea will be infinitely easier if you are fueled by vigor and excitement about this entirely natural and, dare I say, welcome period of no periods.

I certainly do not mourn the monthly pains, the inconvenience of buying expensive and ecologically unfriendly menstrual products (though there are emerging alternatives), and being in charge of contraception. Instead, I'm singing a heavenly (though dew-less) hallelujah for my reprieve from that aspect of my biology. It means that I can concentrate on other priorities.

We need to ensure that society celebrates and accepts women at every stage of their lives. To have a span of years which might exceed our reproductive decades is a precious gift of extra time into which we can pack our ambitions and fulfill our outstanding or newly minted dreams.

Returning to the grandmother hypothesis, the more I think about it, the more I believe modern society is possible only because of the gift of menopause.

What a brilliant way for women's lives to evolve, making our fertility just one era of a full lifespan and celebrating not just our gestating abilities but also our value as mature, confident, and far wiser adults. So let's embrace the positives by ending the negative imagery and investing in better education, support, and opportunities for girls and women as they move through their biological lives. This really is a final frontier when it comes to women reaching their full potential. Educate everybody, offer the right support, and watch society and the economy flourish, in the company of far happier and more fulfilled women.

Yes, menopause is The Change, but one for the better. Watch out for the menopausal woman, for she is driven and passionate, and eager for new and inspiring adventures.

I know that I am bolder, more enterprising, and certainly less insecure than I have ever been. And the evidence points to many women in their fifties becoming equally fearless, ditching bad relationships, embarking on new careers, and reinventing themselves both socially and biologically by adopting healthier lifestyles and emotional resilience for the second phase of their lives.

Renewed confidence is the greatest and perhaps most surprising gift, bearing in mind the bad publicity. It allows you to find peace in your own company, to wear what you like rather than let the vagaries of fashion dictate wardrobe choices, to enjoy more intimate and honest relationships with your friends and family, and to find laughter and wisdom where others see only the tragedy of leaving youth behind. I know nowadays how to wring every last ounce of pleasure from each breathing moment and intend to keep doing so, as healthily and heartily as possible, for as many more decades as my beating heart allows.

As my gender stands taller (though not yet tall enough) and more visible, with women's issues on the menu as never before, it's high time we dragged this last installment of our biological cycle into the daylight where it belongs. Dispelling the negative assumptions about menopause removes the last great barrier to full equality.

By accepting that we can't turn back tides or time, we can focus instead on leading more rewarding and illuminated lifestyles, and so make the most of these promising decades that lie ahead.

Confronting your worst fears can only make you stronger, and that's how my own chapter closes. The aim is an ambitious one, to rebrand menopause as a fresh start and a new phase of life, a second spring, with all the bursting shoots of inspiration and exciting activity that that vision conjures up, rather than seeing your periods stopping as the first nail in a rapidly slamming coffin lid. Thousands of years of counterarguments need to be totally dismissed as we rise like the proverbial phoenix from the ashes of our youth and fertility. Hopefully now you have the knowledge and the tools you need to survive and thrive. It's time for each and every one of us to embrace what lies ahead instead of mourning what we've left behind.

Acknowledgments

The brilliant, witty, and patient Dr. Mary Jane Minkin, who has given so generously of her time, knowledge, and insight. She is an inspiration, and we are both fortunate and grateful to have worked with her.

Melissa Ashley, cofounder, Menopause Mandate US, for her expert help, support, and invaluable suggestions.

Jamie Land, for providing (all!) the women in his life, and Jane Ridley and Sarah Ivens for their time and their networks.

Naomi Watts for her friendship, her unflagging sisterly support, and for being such a brave and pioneering inspiration for so many.

All of our colleagues at Menopause Mandate in the US and the UK who have raised the menopause flag with us and kept it flying since our inception. In particular Laura Biggs, who quite literally powers the machine, and Melissa Robertson, for her award-winning creative ideas.

Varun Chandra, managing partner of Hakluyt, for easing our path into the US.

Our editor Kara Watson for believing in the book; we are so excited to be published in the US, and our agent Natasha Fairweather for securing us not one but two book deals on the hot topic of menopause.

All those who so kindly gave their expertise and stories.

And Dr. Sharon Malone for lending us her great wisdom.

Notes

INTRODUCTION

1 *With around 1.3 million women becoming menopausal every year in the US*: Kimberly Peacock; Karen Carlson; Kari M. Ketvertis; Chaddie Doerr, "Menopause (Nursing)" (updated December 21, 2023), StatPearls [Internet] (Treasure Island, FL: StatPearls Publishing, January 2024). Available from: https://www.ncbi.nlm.nih.gov/books/NBK568694/.

1 *one in four women over the age of forty (around 83 million in total)*: Katie Keating, "1 in 4 Americans is a woman over 40. So why do so many feel ignored?," *fastcompany.com*, July 1, 2021, https://www.fastcompany.com/90649731/1-in-4-americans-is-a-woman-over-40-so-why-do-so-many-feel-ignored.

4 *Dr. Sharon Malone has described it, entering our "third trimester of life"*: Michele Obama, "What Your Mother Never Told You About Health" with Dr. Sharon Malone, September 30, 2020, *The Light Podcast*, 27:55, https://podcasts.apple.com/gb/podcast/what-your-mother-never-told-you-about-health-with-dr/id1532956108?i=1000493064968.

7 *Despite homo sapiens spending over 300,000 years on this planet*: J. P. Rafferty, "Just How Old Is Homo sapiens?," *Encyclopedia Britannica*, June 21, 2017, https://www.britannica.com/story/just-how-old-is-homo-sapiens.

CHAPTER ONE: Pointless and Poisonous: Menopause in the First Millennia

9 *As recently as 1969, the American doctor David Reuben*: David R. Reuben, MD, *Everything You Always Wanted to Know About Sex* (London & New York: Harper-Collins, 1970; first published 1969), 288.

9 *Aristotle managed one nearly accurate bit of detail around 300 BC*: Y. Muscat Baron, "A history of the menopause," Msida: University of Malta, Faculty of Medicine & Surgery, Department of Obstetrics and Gynaecology, 2012, https://www.um.edu.mt/library/oar/handle/123456789/51273.

10 *women contain too much blood due to our coldness, general ineptitude*: Lesley Dean-Jones, "Menstrual Bleeding According to the Hippocratics and Aristotle," *Transactions of the American Philological Association* 119 (1989): 177–91, https://doi.org/10.2307/284268.

10 *A sixth-century physician, Aetius of Amida, suggested that the "very fat cease early"*: Darrel W. Amundsen and Carol Jean Diers, "The Age of Menopause in Medieval Europe," *Human Biology* 45, no. 4 (1973): 605–12, http://www.jstor.org/stable/41459908.

10 *the "first female gynecologist"*: Monica H. Green, "Who, What Is 'Trotula,'" *academia .edu* (February 21, 2023), https://doi.org/10.17613/y0n1 w350.

11 *Then there's Saint Hildegard of Bingen in twelfth-century Germany*: Darrel W. Amundsen and Diers, "The Age of Menopause in Medieval Europe."

11 *The thirteenth-century German philosopher and scientist Albertus Magnus*: Jessica E. Godfrey, *Attitudes Towards Post-Menopausal Women in the High and Late Middle Ages 1100-1400* (Xlibris US, 2011), 30.

12 *The sixteenth-century Italian doctor Giovanni Marinello*: Michael Stolberg, "A Woman's Hell? Medical Perceptions of Menopause in Preindustrial Europe," *Bulletin of the History of Medicine* 73, no. 3 (1999): 404–28, http://www.jstor.org/stable/44445288.

12 *Louise Foxcroft explains that eighty percent of those put to death*: Louise Foxcroft, *Hot Flushes, Cold Science: A History of the Modern Menopause* (London: Granta Books, 2009), 61, 64–67.

13 *the most famous of these took place in Salem, Massachusetts*: Jess Blumberg, "A Brief History of the Salem Witch Trials. One town's strange journey from paranoia to pardon," *Smithsonian Magazine*, October 23, 2007, updated October 24, 2022, https://www.smithsonianmag.com/history/a-brief-history-of-the-salem-witch -trials-175162489/.

13 *The idea that aging equaled a pact with the Devil*: Reginald Scot (edited by Brinsley Nicholson, MD), *The Discoverie of Witchcraft*, edited by Brinsley Nicholson, MD (London: Elliot Stock, 1584, reprinted 1886), https://www.gutenberg.org/files /60766/60766-h/60766-h.htm.

14 *a time during which you were likely to be committed to a psychiatric institution*: Dan Evon, "Reasons for Admission to Insane Asylums in the 19th Century: A list purportedly documents the myriad reasons or symptoms behind patients' being admitted to insane asylums back in the 1800s," snopes.com, February 8, 2016, https://www.snopes.com/fact-check/reasons-admission-insane-asylum-1800s/.

14 *It was a French doctor who coined the word "menopause"*: Alison M. Downham Moore, "The French Elaboration of Ideas about Menopause, Sexuality and Ageing 1805-1920," *French History and Civilization* 8 (2019): 34–50.

14 *may have come up with that fairly bland term*: M. Notelovitz, *The Climacteric in Perspective: Proceedings of the Fourth International Congress on the Menopause, held at Lake Buena Vista, Florida, October 28–November 2, 1984* (Germany: Springer Netherlands, 2012), 125.

14 *"Not only a prisoner of her reproductive functions"*: Carroll Smith-Rosenberg, "Puberty to Menopause: The Cycle of Femininity in Nineteenth-Century America," *Feminist Studies* 1, no. 3/4 (1973): 59, http://www.jstor.org/stable/1566480.

15 *"Insanity frequently occurs at the change of constitution"*: W. Tyler Smith, "The Climacteric Disease in Women; A Paroxysmal Affection Occurring at the Decline of the Catamenia," *London Journal of Medicine* 1, no. 7 (July 1849); 604, https://www .jstor.org/stable/25493754?seq=5.

15 *"There is a predisposition to many diseases"*: Carroll Smith-Rosenberg, "Puberty to Menopause: The Cycle of Femininity in Nineteenth-Century America," *Feminist Studies* 1, no. 3/4 (1973): 65, http://www.jstor.org/stable/1566480.

15 *"There may be a drowsy look"*: E. J. Tilt, *The Change of Life in Health and Disease: A Practical Treatise on the Nervous and Other Affections Incidental to Women at the Decline of Life* (London: John Churchill, 1857).

16 *"My experience teaches me that a marked increase of sexual impulse"*: Carroll Smith-Rosenberg, "Puberty to Menopause: The Cycle of Femininity in Nineteenth-Century America," *Feminist Studies* 1, no. 3/4 (1973): 66, http://www.jstor.org/stable/1566480.

16 *Keep calm and carry on being domesticated*: E. Showalter, *The Female Malady: Women, Madness and English Culture, 1830–1980* (London: Virago, 1987), 123.

16 *"Heavy and prolonged sleep, particularly in the morning"*: W. Tyler Smith, "The Climacteric Disease in Women; A Paroxysmal Affection Occurring at the Decline of the Catamenia," *London Journal of Medicine* 1, no. 7 (1849): 601–9, http://www.jstor.org/stable/25493754.

18 *"seems to correct the toxic influence"*: E. J. Tilt, *The Change of Life in Health and Disease: A Practical Treatise on the Nervous and Other Affections Incidental to Women at the Decline of Life* (United Kingdom: J. Churchill, 1857).

18 *six to eight … leeches on the perineum*: E. J. Tilt, *A Handbook of Uterine Therapeutics and of Diseases of Women* (New York: D Appleton and Company, 1869).

18 *An especially sadistic-sounding expert named Dr. Isaac Baker Brown*: Elizabeth Sheehan, "Victorian Clitoridectomy: Isaac Baker Brown and His Harmless Operative Procedure," *Medical Anthropology Newsletter* 12, no. 4 (1981): 9–15, http://www.jstor.org/stable/647794.

18 *surgeon Andrew Currier advocated simple problem-solving in the 1890s*: Janice Delaney, Mary Jane Lupton, Emily Toth, *The Curse: A Cultural History of Menstruation* (Champaign: University of Illinois Press, 1988), 217, 222

18 *French scientist injected a menopausal patient with ovarian extract*: Frances B. McCrea, "The Politics of Menopause: The 'Discovery' of a Deficiency Disease," *Social Problems* 31, no. 1 (1983): 111–23, https://doi.org/10.2307/800413, 112.

19 *doctors in the States were starting to rebrand menopause*: Judith A. Houck, *Hot and Bothered, Women, Medicine and Menopause in Modern America* (Cambridge: Harvard University Press, 2008), 14–16, 33.

19 *in 1849, Elizabeth Blackwell was the first woman*: Stacey Weiner, "Celebrating 10 women medical pioneers," AAMC News, March 3, 2020, https://www.aamc.org/news/celebrating-10-women-medical-pioneers#:~:text=In%201849%2C%20Elizabeth%20Blackwell%20became,care%20from%20a%20female%20doctor.

19 *During the 1890s there were seventeen*: A. Walling, K. Nilsen, and K. J. Templeton, "The Only Woman in the Room: Oral Histories of Senior Women Physicians in a Midwestern City," *Women's Health Reports* 1, no. 1 (August 31, 2020): 279–86, https://doi.org/10.1089/whr.2020.0041.

20 *Sigmund Freud is perhaps most famous for his early twentieth-century*: Janice Delaney, Mary Jane Upton, Emily Toth, *The Curse: A Cultural History of Menstruation* (Champaign: University of Illinois Press, 1988), 220.

20 *A student of Freud's, the psychiatrist Helene Deutsch*: Joan C. Callahan, *"Menopause, A Midlife Passage"* (Bloomington: Indiana University Press, 1993), 51.

21 *"Because of menopause, m'lud"*: Phyllis T. Bookspan and Maxine Kline, "On Mirror and Gavels. A Chronicle of How Menopause Was Used as a Legal Defense Against Women," *Indiana Law Review* 32, no. 1267 (1999), https://mckinneylaw.iu.edu /practice/law-reviews/ilr/pdf/vol32p1267.pdf.

21 *Famous feminist Simone de Beauvoir was also pretty mournful*: Simone de Beauvoir, *The Second Sex* (Vintage Digital, 2014, first published 1949).

21 *"It has been far less somber"*: Simon de Beauvoir, *All Said and Done* (Paragon House, New York, 1993, First published 1972) https://archive.org/details/isbn _9781569249819/page/n5/mode/2up?q=joy+of+loving.

21 *In the swinging sixties, MHT was all the rage*: Robert A. Wilson, *Feminine Forever* (London: W. H. Allen, 1966), 30.

22 *"Even today the literature . . . defines menopause"*: Frances B. McCrea, "The Politics of Menopause: The 'Discovery' of a Deficiency Disease," *Social Problems* 31, no. 1 (1983): 111–23, https://doi.org/10.2307/800413, 112.

23 *Phyllis Kernoff Mansfield, professor emeritus of women's studies*: Nancy Marie Brown, "A Natural History of Menopause," Pennsylvania State University, April 30, 1998, https://www.psu.edu/news/research/story/natural-history-menopause/.

26 *more likely to experience an adverse drug reaction*: H. Whitley and W. Lindsey, "Sex-based differences in drug activity," *American Family Physician* 80, no. 11 (December 1, 2009): 1254–58, https://pubmed.ncbi.nlm.nih.gov/19961138/.

26 *lists the physiological differences between the sexes*: A. Holdcroft, "Gender bias in research: How does it affect evidence based medicine?," *Journal of the Royal Society of Medicine* 100, no.1 (January 2007): 2–3, https://doi.org/10.1177/01410 7680710000102.

26 *Women's pain is less understood*: Professor Amanda Williams, "Analysis: Women's pain is routinely underestimated, and gender stereotypes are to blame," University College London, Department of Clinical, Education and Health Psychology, April 9, 2021, https://www.ucl.ac.uk/news/2021/apr/analysis-womens-pain -routinely-underestimated-and-gender-stereotypes-are-blame.

CHAPTER TWO: A Road Map to Menopause

30 *oldest recorded menopause*: Janice Delaney, Mary Jane Lupton, Emily Toth, *The Curse: A Cultural History of Menstruation* (Champaign: University of Illinois Press, 1988), 214.

30 *now starting to be recognized that Latinas and Black women*: "Exclusion of Black and Hispanic women from health studies masked racial disparities on menopausal aging," Michigan School of Public Health, June 29, 2023, https://sph.umich.edu /news/2023posts/racial-disparities-menopausal-aging-masked-exclusion-early -menopausal-women-womens-health-study.html.

31 *giraffes spend thirty percent of their lives*: Zoe Muller and Stephen Harris, "A review of the social behaviour of the giraffe *Giraffa camelopardalis*: A misunderstood but socially complex species," *Mammal Review* 52, no. 1 (January 2022), https://online library.wiley.com/doi/full/10.1111/mam.12268.

31 *"a defect in the evolution of human beings"*: David R. Reuben, MD, *Everything You Always Wanted to Know About Sex* (London & New York: 1970; New York: David McKay, 1969), 284.

32 *maximum human lifespan hasn't changed*: J. P. Griffin, "Changing life expectancy throughout history," *Letter to the Journal of the Royal Society of Medicine* 101, no. 12 (December 1, 2008): 577, https://doi.org/10.1258/jrsm.2008.08k037.

32 *From 1500 to 1800, early church records in the UK*: Lynda Payne, "Health in England (16th–18th c.)," in Children and Youth in History, Item #166, https://chnm.gmu .edu/cyh/teaching-modules/166.html (accessed August 10, 2021).

32 *more than a third of women are said to have died*: Sarah Bryson, "Childbirth in Medieval and Tudor Times," The Tudor Society, 2016. https://www.tudorsociety .com/childbirth-in-medieval-and-tudor-times-by-sarah-bryson/?noamp =mobile#comments.

32 *infant mortality could be up to sixty times*: Russell W. Currier and John A. Widness, "A Brief History of Milk Hygiene and Its Impact on Infant Mortality from 1875 to 1925 and Implications for Today: A Review," *Journal of Food Protection* 81, no. 10 (October 1, 2018): 1713–22, https://doi.org/10.4315/0362-028X.JFP-18-186.

32 *Professor Kristen Hawkes's work on the subject*: K. Hawkes, J. F. O'Connell, and N. G. Blurton Jones, "Hardworking Hadza grandmothers," in *Comparative Socioecology: The Behavioural Ecology of Humans and Other Mammals*, edited by V. Standen and R. A. Foley (London: Basil Blackwell, June 1989): 341–66, http://content.csbs.utah .edu/~hawkes/Hawkes_al89ha.

33 *"Men's foraging was not consistent"*: J. F. O'Connell, K. Hawkes, and N. Blurton Jones, "Hadza men's follows, 1985–1986: Data and implications for ideas about ancestral male foraging effort in human evolution," *PaleoAnthropology* 2024, no. 1 (May 1, 2024): 112–38, https://paleoanthropology.org/ojs/index.php/paleo/article/view /1084.

34 *In 2012, Hawkes published a paper with a mathematical simulation*: K. Hawkes, P. S. Kim, and J. E. Coxworth, "Increased Longevity Evolves from Grandmothering," *Proceeding of the Royal Society* 279, no. 1749 (December 22, 2012), https:// doi.org/10.1098/rspb.2012.1751.

36 *A 2023 nationwide assessment revealed*: Jennifer T. Allen, Shahar Laks, Carolyn Zahler-Miller, Bunja J. Rungruang, Kelli Braun, Steven R. Goldstein, Peter F. Schnatz, "Needs assessment of menopause education in United States obstetrics and gynecology residency training programs," *Menopause* 30, no. 10 (October 2023): 1002–1005, https://doi.org/10.1097/GME.0000000000002234.

36 *A 2019 Mayo Clinic survey*: Juliana M. Kling, MD, MPH; Kathy L. MacLaughlin, MD; Peter F. Schnatz, DO; Kristin Mara, MS; Karla S. Fohmader Hilsaca, PhD; Stephanie S. Faubion, MD, "Menopause Management Knowledge in Postgraduate Family Medicine, Internal Medicine, and Obstetrics and Gynecology Residents: A Cross-Sectional Survey, *Mayo Clinic Proceedings* 94, no. 2 (February 2019): 242–53, https://doi.org/10.1016/j.mayocp.2018.08.033.

36 *In 2022, Stephanie S. Faubion*: S. S. Faubion and C. Shufelt, "The Menopause Man-

agement Vacuum," *The Cancer Journal* 28, no. 3 (May/June 2022): 191–95, https://doi.org/10.1097/PPO.0000000000000594.

37 *And how does this on-paper bedlam translate*: Jennifer Wolff, "What Doctors Don't Know About Menopause. Three out of four women who seek help for symptoms don't receive it," AARP Magazine, July 20, 2018, https://www.aarp.org/health/conditions-treatments/info-2018/menopause-symptoms-doctors-relief-treatment.html.

37 *An appalling one in ten women in the US*: "Women's Health Insurance Coverage," KFF Women's Health Policy, December 13, 2023, https://www.kff.org/womens-health-policy/fact-sheet/womens-health-insurance-coverage/.

37 *women aged from forty-four to sixty*: Stephanie S. Faubion, MD, MBA; Felicity Enders, PhD; Mary S. Hedges, MD; Kristin Mara, MS; Joan M. Griffin, PhD; Ekta Kapoor, MBBS, "Impact of Menopause Symptoms on Women in the Workplace," *Mayo Clinic Proceedings* 98, no. 6 (April 26, 2023): 833–45, https://doi.org/10.1016/j.mayocp.2023.02.025.

40 *"any time you're dealing with a specifically gendered dimension"*: E. A. Paine, D. Umberson, and C. Reczek, "Sex in Midlife: Women's Sexual Experiences in Lesbian and Straight Marriages," *Journal of Marriage and the Family* 98, no. 6 (July 2, 2018): 7–23, https://doi.org/10.1111/jomf.12508.

42 *SWAN women were born between 1944 and 1954*: S. D. Harlow, S-A. M. Burnett-Bowie, G. A. Greendale et al., "Disparities in Reproductive Aging and Midlife Health between Black and White Women: The Study of Women's Health Across the Nation (SWAN)," *Women's Midlife Health* 8, no. 3 (February 8, 2022), https://doi.org/10.1186/s40695-022-00073-y.

42 *Another SWAN paper about hot flashes*: Nancy E. Avis, Sybil L. Crawford, Gail Greendale et al., "Duration of menopausal vasomotor symptoms over the menopause transition," *JAMA Internal Medicine* 175, no. 4(April 2015): 531–39, https://doi.org/10.1001/jamainternmed.2014.8063.

43 *Latina and non-Latina Black women experience*: Yamnia I. Cortés and Valentina Marginean, "Key factors in menopause health disparities and inequities: Beyond race and ethnicity," *Current Opinion in Endocrine and Metabolic Research* 26 (October 2022), https://doi.org/10.1016/j.coemr.2022.100389; https://www.sciencedirect.com/science/article/pii/S2451965022000746.

43 *Vaginal dryness was present in thirty to forty percent*: Robin Green and Nanette Santoro, "Menopausal symptoms and ethnicity: The Study of Women's Health Across the Nation," *Women's Health* (March 1, 2009): 127–33, https://doi.org/10.2217/17455057.5.2.127.

43 *There's insufficient research into Asian American women*: Alisha Haridasani Gupta, "How Menopause Affects Women of Color," *New York Times*, updated September 4, 2023, https://www.nytimes.com/2023/08/23/well/live/menopause-symptoms-women-of-color.html.

43 *little research into the experiences of Native American women*: S. D. Reed, J. W. Lampe, C. Qu, W. K. Copeland, G. Gundersen, S. Fuller, and K. M. Newton, "Premenopausal vasomotor symptoms in an ethnically diverse population," *Meno-*

pause (February 2014): 153–58, https://doi.org/10.1097/GME.0b013e318295
2228.

43 *A 2023 study looking at almost 66,000 women*: Celeste Krewson, "Significant racial disparities seen in hormone therapy prescription," Contemporary OB/GYN, September 27, 2023, https://www.contemporaryobgyn.net/view/significant-racial-disparities-seen-in-hormone-therapy-prescription.

43 *In a 2022 analysis of SWAN data*: P. S. David and J. M. Kling, "Moving toward health equity: The influence of race and ethnicity on choice and quality of life of menopause treatment in midlife women," *Menopause* 29, no. 12 (December 1, 2022): 1353–54, https://pubmed.ncbi.nlm.nih.gov/36346986/.

44 *effects of* Roe vs Wade *are cascading*: J. A. Berg and N. F. Woods, "Overturning *Roe v. Wade*: Consequences for midlife women's health and well-being," *Women's Midlife Health* 9, no. 2 (January 6, 2023): 2, https://doi.org/10.1186/s40695-022-00085-8.

45 *In 2023, President Joe Biden*: The White House Initiative on Women's Health Research, February 21, 2024 (launched 2023), https://www.whitehouse.gov/white-house-initiative-on-womens-health-research/.

45 *On March 7, 2024, in the State of the Union address*: President Joe Biden, "Executive Order on Advancing Women's Health Research and Innovation," March 18, 2024, https://www.whitehouse.gov/briefing-room/presidential-actions/2024/03/18/executive-order-on-advancing-womens-health-research-and-innovation/.

45 *Halle Berry, who was memorably . . . misdiagnosed*: Dan Diamond, "Senators, Halle Berry unveil $275 million bill to boost menopause care," *Washington Post*, May 2, 2024, https://www.washingtonpost.com/health/2024/05/02/menopause-congress-halle-berry/.

46 *only around ten percent of the NIH's current budget*: Sharon Malone, M.D., and Jennifer Weiss-Wolf, "A Menopause Research Bill Reaches Congress," Oprah Daily, updated December 14, 2023, https://www.oprahdaily.com/life/health/a45549121/menopause-research-congressional-bill/.

CHAPTER THREE: First Impact

57 *ninety-one percent of women recorded between one and three occurrences*: S. D. Harlow and P. Paramsothy, "Menstruation and the menopausal transition," *Obstetrics and Gynecology Clinics of North America* 38, no. 3 (September 2011): 595–607, https://doi.org/10.1016/j.ogc.2011.05.010.

58 *over seventy percent of women*: K. Peacock, K. Carlson, K. M. Ketvertis, C. Doerr, "Menopause (Nursing)" (updated December 21, 2023), StatPearls [Internet] (Treasure Island, FL: StatPearls Publishing, January 2024). Available from: https://www.ncbi.nlm.nih.gov/books/NBK568694/.

59 *seventy percent of perimenopausal women*: L. Born, G. Koren, E. Lin, and M. Steiner, "A new, female-specific irritability rating scale," *Journal of Psychiatry and Neuroscience* 33, no. 4 (July 2008): 344–54. https://www.ncbi.nlm.nih.gov/pmc/articles/PMC2440789/.

60 *eighty percent of us may get them*: Ramandeep Bansal and Neelam Aggarwal,

"Menopausal Hot Flashes: A Concise Review," *Journal of Mid-Life Health* 10, no. 1 (January–March 2019): 6–13, https://www.ncbi.nlm.nih.gov/pmc/articles /PMC6459071/.

60 *for around twenty percent, they can be disruptive*: Reviewed by Wen Shen, MD, "Did I Just Have a Hot Flash? I'm 44!," Johns Hopkins Medicine, https://www.hopkins medicine.org/health/wellness-and-prevention/did-i-just-have-a-hot-flash-im -44#:~:text=For%2010%20to%2015%20percent,to%20speak%20with%20your%20 gynecologist.

62 *women in the first year postmenopause*: M. T. Weber, L. H. Rubin, and P. M. Maki, "Cognition in perimenopause: The effect of transition stage," *Menopause* 20, no. 5 (May 2013): 511–17, https://doi.org/10.1097/gme.0b013e31827655e5.

64 *We know that brain chemistry can affect mood*: Paraskevi Vivien Rekkas, Alan A. Wilson, Vivian Wai Han Lee, et al, "Greater monoamine oxidase a binding in peri-menopausal age as measured with carbon 11-labeled harmine positron emission tomography," *JAMA Psychiatry* 71, no. 8 (August 2014): 873–79, https://doi.org /10.1001/jamapsychiatry.2014.250.

64 *suicide rates are consistently highest in women*: Preeti Vankar, "Female suicide rate in the U.S. from 2001 to 2021, by age group," Statista, March 4, 2024, https://www .statista.com/statistics/1114127/female-suicide-rate-in-the-us-by-age-group/.

CHAPTER FOUR: MHT, Part One

75 *Back in 2002 the results of a major study*: "NHLBI stops trial of estrogen plus pro-gestin due to increased breast cancer risk and lack of overall benefit," *Southern Medical Journal* 95, no. 8 (August 2002): 795–97, https://pubmed.ncbi.nlm.nih.gov /12190211/.

75 *In May 2024, a twenty-year follow-up revealed*: JoAnn E. Manson, MD, DrPH; Rowan T. Chlebowski, MD, PhD; Marcia L. Stefanick, PhD et al., "Menopausal Hormone Therapy and Health Outcomes During the Intervention and Extended Post-stopping Phases of the Women's Health Initiative Randomized Trials," *JAMA* 310, no. 13 (October 2, 2013): 1353–68, DOI 10.1001/jama.2013.278040; https:// jamanetwork.com/journals/jama/fullarticle/1745676.

76 *The "modern theory of menstruation"*: Sahar M. Stephens and Kelle H. Moley, "Follicular origins of modern reproductive endocrinology," *American Journal of Physiology Endocrinology and Metabolism* 297, no. 6 (December 2009): E1235–36, https://journals.physiology.org/doi/full/10.1152/ajpendo.00575.2009.

77 *a word coined in 1905 by Ernest Starling*: J. R. Tata, "One hundred years of hor-mones," *EMBO Reports* 6 (June 1, 2005): 490–96, https://doi.org/10.1038/sj.em bor.7400444.

77 *A trio of men isolated and purified estrogen*: James Woods, MD, and Elizabeth Warner, MD, "The History of Estrogen," Obstetrics & GYnecology: meno-Pause (blog), February 17, 2016, https://www.urmc.rochester.edu/ob-gyn/ur -medicine-menopause-and-womens-health/menopause-blog/february-2016 /the-history-of-estrogen.aspx#:~:text=Then%2C%20in%201906%2C%20 secretions%20from,and%20gennan%20(to%20produce).

77 *crystalline progesterone was isolated*: Colleen L Casey and Christine A Murray, "HT update: spotlight on estradiol/norethindrone acetate combination therapy," *Clinical Interventions in Aging* 3, no. 1 (2008): 9–16, https://www.readcube.com/articles /10.2147%2Fcia.s1663; https://pubmed.ncbi.nlm.nih.gov/18488874/.

77 *the production of a substance called Emmenin*: Meryl Davids Landau, "The Wild History of Women's Hormone Therapy," Everyday Health, updated December 13, 2022, https://www.everydayhealth.com/womens-health/hormones/history-hormone -therapy/.

78 *In the early 1940s, the resulting drug, Premarin*: Stephen K. Ritter, "Premarin, Purpose Hormone," *C&EN ACS* 83, no. 25 (June 20, 2005), https://cen.acs.org/articles /83/i25/Premarin.html#:~:text=Premarin%20was%20introduced%20in%20 1941,derived%20from%20pregnant%20mare's%20urine.

78 *by the mid-1970s, estrogen was the fifth*: G. E. Kohn, K. M. Rodriguez, J. Hotaling, and A. W. Pastuszak, "The History of Estrogen Therapy," *SexualMedicine Reviews* 7. no. 3 (July 2019): 416–21, https://doi.org/10.1016/j.sxmr.2019.03.006.

78 *Premarin was the number one prescribed drug*: Bloomberg News, "FDA Allows American Home to Retain Its Monopoly on a Drug" *New York Times*, May 6, 1997, https://timesmachine.nytimes.com/timesmachine/1997/05/06/960560.html ?pageNumber=74.

79 *one of the principal investigators in the WHI study*: R. D. Langer, "The evidence base for HRT: What can we believe?," *Climacteric* 20, no. 2 (March 10, 2017): 91, https:// doi.org/10.1080/13697137.2017.1280251.

81 *Use of MHT plummeted by around eighty percent*: J. E. Manson, J. E. and A. M. Kaunitz, "Menopause Management—Getting Clinical Care Back on Track," *New England Journal of Medicine* 374, no. 9 (March 3, 2016): 803–806, https://doi.org /10.1056/NEJMp1514242.

81 *a 2013 study of OB/GYN residency programs*: M. S. Christianson, J. A. Ducie, K. Altman, A. M. Khafagy, and W. Shen, "Menopause education: Needs assessment of American obstetrics and gynecology residents," *Menopause* 20, no. 11 (November 2013): 1120–25, https://doi.org/10.1097/GME.0b013e31828ced7f.

81 *A poll in 2023, despite all the myth-busting*: Celeste Krewson, "Survey shows menopause curriculums lacking in residency programs," Contemporary OB/GYN, August 11, 2023, https://www.contemporaryobgyn.net/view/survey-shows-meno pause-curriculums-lacking-in-residency-programs.

82 *I was over the moon when a twenty-year follow-up*: J. E. Manson, C. J. Crandall, J. E. Rossouw et al. "The Women's Health Initiative Randomized Trials and Clinical Practice: A Review," *JAMA* 331, no. 20 (May 28, 2024): 1748–60, https://doi.org/10 .1001/jama.2024.6542.

82 *the* Washington Post *covered it*: Marlene Cimons, "No need to fear menopause hormone drugs, finds major women's health study," *Washington Post*, May 1, 2024, https://www.washingtonpost.com/wellness/2024/05/01/menopause-hormones -hrt-safety-whi/.

83 *MHT use remains shockingly low*: Sophie Putka, "Hormone Therapy Use For Menopause Has Remained Low Since 2007," Medpagetoday, September 13, 2024,

https://www.medpagetoday.com/meetingcoverage/tms/111948?xid=nl_mpt_
confroundup_2024-09-18&mh=610980f77e849f799416940be6456822.

85 *In a 2017 Mayo Clinic survey:* Juliana M. Kling, MD, MPH; Kathy L. MacLaughlin, MD; Peter F. Schnatz, DO; Kristin Mara, MS; Karla S. Fohmader Hilsaca, PhD; and Stephanie S. Faubion, MD, "Menopause Management Knowledge in Postgraduate Family Medicine, Internal Medicine, and Obstetrics and Gynecology Residents: A Cross-Sectional Survey," *Mayo Clinic Proceedings* 94, no. 2 (February 2019), https://doi.org/10.1016/j.mayocp.2018.08.033.

85 *Let's also remember that there are women dying:* Philip M. Sarrel, MD; Valentine Y. Njike, MD, MPH; Valentina Vinante, MD; and David L. Katz, MD, MPH, "The mortality toll of estrogen avoidance: An analysis of excess deaths among hysterectomized women aged 50 to 59 years," *American Journal of Public Health* 103, no. 9 (August 7, 2013): 1583–88, https://doi.org/10.2105/AJPH.2013.301295.

CHAPTER FOUR: MHT, Part Two

100 *According to the CDC, over 60 million women:* "About Women and Heart Disease," CDC Heart Disease, May 15, 2024, https://www.cdc.gov/heart-disease/about/women-and-heart-disease.html#:~:text=Overview,affect%20women%20at%20any%20age.

100 *Women are far more likely to develop coronary heart disease:* Laura Williamson, "The connection between menopause and cardiovascular disease risks," American Heart Association, February 20, 2023, https://www.heart.org/en/news/2023/02/20/the-connection-between-menopause-and-cardiovascular-disease-risks.

101 *women fare worse after heart attacks:* Office on Women's Health, "Heart attack and women," womenshealth.gov, last updated February 17, 2021, https://www.womenshealth.gov/heart-disease-and-stroke/heart-disease/heart-attack-and-women.

101 *approximately 10 million Americans have osteoporosis:* Bone Health and Osteoporosis Foundation, "What Women Need to Know," https://www.bonehealthandosteoporosis.org/preventing-fractures/general-facts/what-women-need-to-know/#:~:text=How%20fast%20you%20lose%20bone,greater%20chance%20of%20developing%20osteoporosis.

102 *those using estrogen-only MHT in midlife to treat menopause symptoms:* M. Nerattini, S. Jett, C. Andy, C. Carlton, C. Zarate, C. Boneu, M. Battista, S. Pahlajani, S. Loeb-Zeitlin, Y. Havryulik, S. Williams, P. Christos, M. Fink, R. D. Brinton, and L. Mosconi, "Systematic review and meta-analysis of the effects of menopause hormone therapy on risk of Alzheimer's disease and dementia," *Frontiers in Aging Neuroscience* 15 (October 23, 2023): 1260427, https://doi.org/10.3389/fnagi.2023.1260427.

CHAPTER FIVE: A Literal "Pause"

112 *A 2007 study conducted in Ecuador:* Patricia Leon, Peter Chedraui, Luis Hidalgo, Fernando Ortiz, "Perceptions and attitudes toward the menopause among middle aged women from Guayaquil, Ecuador," *Maturitas* 57, no. 3 (February 2, 2007): 233–38, https://doi.org/10.1016/j.maturitas.2007.01.003.

112 *In taped interviews in Jordan in 2008:* A. I. Mahadeen, RN, PhD; J. O. Halabi, RN,

PhD; L. C. Callister, RN, PhD, Faan, "Menopause: A qualitative study of Jordanian women's perceptions," *International Nursing Review* 55, no. 4 (November 11, 2008): 427–33, https://doi.org/10.1111/j.1466-7657.2008.00662.x.

112 *anthropologist called Marcha Flint noted*: Marcha Flint, "The menopause: Reward or punishment?," *Psychosomatics: Journal of Consultation and Liaison Psychiatry* 16, no. 4 (October 1975): 161–63, https://doi.org/10.1016/S0033-3182(75)71183-0.

112 *a massive 2015 study led by Dr. Minkin*: Mary Jane Minkin, MD, NCMP; Suzanne Reiter, RNC, NP, MM, MS; and Ricardo Maamari, MD, NCMP, "Prevalence of post-menopausal symptoms in North America and Europe," *Menopause* 22, no. 11 (November, 2015): 1231–38, https://doi.org/10.1097/GME.0000000000000464.

113 *A 2012 study explained that the language used around*: Emma K. Jones, Janelle R. Jurgenson, Judith M. Katzenellenbogen, and Sandra C. Thompson, "Menopause and the influence of culture: another gap for Indigenous Australian women?," *BMC Women's Health* 12, no. 43 (December 12, 2012), https://doi.org/10.1186/1472-6874-12-43.

115 *The 2023 Menopause Society non-hormone therapy position*: NAMS Position Statement: The 2023 nonhormone therapy position statement of The North American Menopause Society, *Menopause: The Journal of the North American Menopause Society* 30, no. 6 (March 21, 2023): 573–90, https://doi.org/10.1097/GME.0000000000002200.

118 *when women are stressed, we release oxytocin*: S. E. Taylor, L. C. Klein, B. P. Lewis, T. L. Gruenewald, R. A. Gurung, and J. A. Updegraff, "Biobehavioral responses to stress in females: Tend-and-befriend, not fight-or-flight," *Psychological review* 107, no. 3 (2000): 411–29, https://doi.org/10.1037/0033-295x.107.3.411.

119 *women who meditated at least once a week for six months*: Min-Kyu Sung, MS; Ul Soon Lee, MA; Na Hyun MD[c] Ha; Eugene Koh, PhD; Hyun-Jeong Yang, PhD, "A potential association of meditation with menopausal symptoms and blood chemistry in healthy women: A pilot cross-sectional study," *Medicine* 99, no. 36 (September 2, 2020): e22048, https://doi.org/10.1097/MD.0000000000022048.

122 *good evidence for tapping and menopause symptoms*: Asieh Mehdipour, Parvin Abedi, Somayeh Ansari, and Maryam Dastoorpoor, "The effectiveness of emotional freedom techniques (EFT) on depression of postmenopausal women: A randomized controlled trial," *Journal of Complementary and Integrative Medicine* 19, no. 3 (May 19, 2021): 737–42, https://doi.org/10.1515/jcim-2020-0245.

CHAPTER SIX: Meno a-Go-Go

128 *I discovered that lethargy can*: Jung Ha Park, Ji Hyun Moon, Hyeon Ju Kim, Mi Hee Kong, Yun Hwan Oh, "Sedentary Lifestyle: Overview of Updated Evidence of Potential Health Risks," *Korean Journal of Family Medicine* 41, no. 6 (November 19, 2020): 365–73, https://doi.org/10.4082/kjfm.20.0165.

130 *In 1979, in the UK, the official drinking advice*: Christopher Snowdon, "The great alcohol cover-up: How public health hid the truth about drinking," *The Spectator*, November 17, 2020, https://www.spectator.co.uk/article/the-great-alcohol-cover-up-how-public-health-hid-the-truth-about-drinking/#:~:text='%20It%20varies%20so%20much%20over,this%20time%20to%2014%20units.

131 *it's recommended that women of legal drinking age*: "About moderate alcohol use," CDC, May 15, 2024, https://www.cdc.gov/alcohol/about-alcohol-use/moderate -alcohol-use.html#:~:text=For%20men%E2%80%94two%20drinks%20or,or%20 less%20in%20a%20day.

133 *The 2020–2025 dietary guidelines for Americans*: Dietary Guidelines for Americans, 2020–2025, "Make Every Bite Count with the Dietary Guidelines," December 2020, https://www.dietaryguidelines.gov/sites/default/files/2020-12/Dietary _Guidelines_for_Americans_2020-2025.pdf.

134 *around two years before your last period*: Gail A. Greendale, Barbara Sternfeld, Mei-Hua Huang, Weijuan Han, Carrie Karvonen-Gutierrez, Kristine Ruppert, Jane A. Cauley, Joel S. Finkelstein, Sheng-Fang Jiang, and Arun S. Karlamangla, "Changes in body composition and weight during the menopause transition," *JCI insight* 4, no. 5 (March 7, 2019): e124865, https://doi.org/10.1172/jci.insight.124865.

134 *The British Menopause Society points out*: "Menopause: Nutrition and Weight Gain," British Menopause Society, June, 2023, https://thebms.org.uk/wp-content/up loads/2023/06/19-BMS-TfC-Menopause-Nutrition-and-Weight-Gain-JUNE2023 -A.pdf.

135 *What's more, diets just don't work*: S. Towers, S. Cole, E. Iboi, C. Montalvo, M.G. Navas-Zuloagam, J.A.M. Pringle, D. Saha, M. Thakur, J. Velazquez-Molina, A. Murillo, C. Castillo-Chavez, and J.C. Norcross, "How long do people stick to a diet resolution? A digital epidemiological estimation of weight loss diet persistence," *Public Health Nutrition* 23, no. 18 (December 14, 2020): 3257–68, https://doi.org /10.1017/S1368980020001597.

136 *This is a combination of the Mediterranean diet and the DASH diet*: Martha Clare Morris, Christy C. Tangney, Yamin Wang, Frank M. Sacks, David A. Bennett, and Neelum T. Aggarwal, "MIND diet associated with reduced incidence of Alzheimer's disease," *Alzheimer's & Dementia: The Journal of the Alzheimer's Association* 11, no. 9 (February 11, 2015): 1007–14, https://doi.org/10.1016/j.jalz.2014.11.009.

137 *Most of us aren't eating enough protein*: "Are you getting too much protein?," Mayo Clinic Press, July 15, 2022, https://mcpress.mayoclinic.org/nutrition-fitness/are -you-getting-too-much-protein/#:~:text=Once%20you%20reach%20ages%20 40,for%20a%2075%2Dkilogram%20person.

137 *Overconsumption of refined sugar*: "How Much Sugar Is Too Much?," American Heart Association, last reviewed May 23, 2024, https://www.heart.org/en/healthy -living/healthy-eating/eat-smart/sugar/how-much-sugar-is-too-much#:~:text =American%20adults%20consume%20an%20average,%2Dpound%20bowling%20 balls%2C%20folks.

138 *By increasing fruit and vegetable intake*: Gerrie-Cor M. Herber-Gast and Gita D. Mishra, "Fruit, Mediterranean-style, and high-fat and -sugar diets are associated with the risk of night sweats and hot flushes in midlife: Results from a prospective cohort study," *American Journal of Clinical Nutrition* 97, no. 5 (May 2013): 1092–1099, https://ajcn.nutrition.org/article/S0002-9165(23)05518-1/fulltext.

138 *Soy also contains protein, fiber, iron, and zinc*: "Soy-rich foods like tofu may help lower heart disease risk," American Heart Association News, March 23, 2020,

https://www.heart.org/en/news/2020/03/23/soy-rich-foods-like-tofu-may-help
-lower-heart-disease-risk.

139 *You might be wondering about the gut microbiome*: Kate M. Bermingham, Inbar
Linenberg, Wendy L. Hall, Kirstin Kadé, Paul W. Franks, Richard Davies et al.,
"Menopause is associated with postprandial metabolism, metabolic health and
lifestyle: The ZOE PREDICT study," *Lancet* 85, no. 104303 (October 18, 2022),
https://doi.org/10.1016/j.ebiom.2022.104303.

139 *And finally, to weight-loss injections or GLP-1 agonists*: Deidre McPhillips, "CNN
Exclusive: Prescriptions for popular diabetes and weight-loss drugs soared, but
access is limited for some patients," CNN, updated September 27, 2023, https://
edition.cnn.com/2023/09/27/health/semaglutide-equitable-access/index.html.

CHAPTER SEVEN: The Hell of Hormonal Insomnia

152 *perimenopausal women were more likely to sleep less than seven hours in a twenty-
four-hour period*: Anjel Vahratian, PhD, "Sleep Duration and Quality Among
Women Aged 40–59, by Menopausal Status," National Health Interview Survey,
2017, https://www.cdc.gov/nchs/data/databriefs/db286.pdf.

152 *it's generally reported that around sixty percent of women*: Louisa McGillicuddy,
"The gender sleep gap: our new survey reveals why women can't sleep," *The
Sunday Times* (London), April 21, 2019, https://www.thetimes.com/life-style
/health-fitness/article/the-gender-sleep-gap-our-new-survey-reveals-why
-women-cant-sleep-jqk3729lv.

153 *Those who sleep fewer than six hours a night*: Marco Hafner, Martin Stepanek, Jirka
Taylor, Wendy M. Troxel, Christian Van Stolk, "Why Sleep Matters: Quantifying
the Economic Costs of Insufficient Sleep. A cross-country comparative analysis," RAND Corporation, November 30, 2016, https://www.rand.org/randeurope
/research/projects/2016/the-value-of-the-sleep-economy.html#:~:text=An%20
individual%20that%20sleeps%20on,are%20associated%20with%20shorter%20
sleep. Lucy Bryan and Dr. Alyssa Dweck, "How Can Menopause Affect Sleep?,"
Sleep Foundation, updated January 18, 2024, https://www.sleepfoundation.org
/women-sleep/menopause-and-sleep.

155 *forty-seven to sixty-seven percent of postmenopausal women*: Shazia Jehan, Evan
Auguste, Ferdinand Zizi et al., "Obstructive Sleep Apnea: Women's Perspective,"
Journal of Sleep Medicine and Disorders 3, no. 6 (August 25, 2016): 1064, https://
www.ncbi.nlm.nih.gov/pmc/articles/PMC5323064/.

155 *The effects of estrogen are vital for the health of the urethra*: Holly J. Jones, Alison J.
Huang, Leslee L. Subak, Jeanette S. Brown, and Kathryn A. Lee, "Bladder Symptoms
in the Early Menopausal Transition," *Journal of Women's Health* 25, no. 5 (May 11,
2016): 457–63, https://www.ncbi.nlm.nih.gov/pmc/articles/PMC4876519/.

158 *About forty percent of adult men are habitual snorers*: (Reviewed by) Imran Shaikh,
MD, and Seema Khosla, MD, "What Is Snoring?," AASM: Sleep Education, November 2020, https://sleepeducation.org/sleep-disorders/snoring/#what-is-snoring.

160 *Our evolutionary adaptation can't keep up*: Aatif Sulleyman, "Netflix's biggest competition is sleep, says CEO Reed Hastings," Independent, April 19, 2017, https://

www.independent.co.uk/tech/netflix-downloads-sleep-biggest-competition
-video-streaming-ceo-reed-hastings-amazon-prime-sky-go-now-tv-a7690561
.html.

163 *A Sleep Foundation survey in 2022 found*: Brianna Graham, "How Much Melatonin Do
We Really Take?," Sleep Foundation, October 20, 2022, https://www.sleepfoundation
.org/sleep-news/how-much-melatonin-do-adults-really-take#:~:text=According%20
to%20a%20separate%20SleepFoundation,melatonin%20to%20fall%20asleep%20
faster.

CHAPTER EIGHT: Women-Shaped Spaces

168 *almost one in five women has left*: "Biote 2022 Women in the Workplace Survey,"
Biote, 2022, https://biote.com/wp-content/uploads/2022/05/Biote-Women-in
-the-Workplace-Survey-Whitepaper.pdf.

169 *sixty percent of US women said they think menopause is generally stigmatized*:
"Break Through The Stigma: Menopause in the Workplace Methodology," Bank of
American Newsroom, June 1, 2023, https://newsroom.bankofamerica.com/con
tent/newsroom/press-releases/2023/06/bofa-report-finds-64--of-women-want
-menopause-specific-benefits-.html.

172 *The US Bureau of Labor Statistics reports that 41 million women*: Caroline Castrillon,
"Why It's Time to Address Menopause in the Workplace," Forbes, March 22, 2023,
https://www.forbes.com/sites/carolinecastrillon/2023/03/22/why-its-time-to
-address-menopause-in-the-workplace/?sh=64589af01f72.

172 *I was mighty jealous when Icelandic women actually did it*: Egill Bjarnason, "Women
across Iceland, including the prime minister, go on strike for equal pay and no
more violence," Associated Press, October 24, 2023, https://apnews.com/article
/iceland-women-strike-equal-pay-970669466116a2b1a5673a8737089d46.

172 *A 2023 Mayo clinic study of 4,440 women*: Stephanie S. Faubion, MD, MBA; Felicity
Enders, PhD; Mary S. Hedges, MD; Kristin Mara, MS; Joan M. Griffin, PhD; Ekta
Kapoor, MBBS, "Impact of Menopause Symptoms on Women in the Workplace,"
Mayo Clinic Proceedings 98, no. 6 (April 2, 2023): 833–45, https://doi.org/10.1016
/j.mayocp.2023.02.025.

173 *In a recent survey, just fifteen percent of large organizations*: Christy Ewing and Co-
rina Leu, "Employers are taking meaningful steps to provide menopause benefits,"
Mercer, October 19, 2023, https://www.mercer.com/en-us/insights/us-health
-news/employers-are-taking-meaningful-steps/#:~:text=The%20percentage%20
of%20large%20organizations,a%20survey%20conducted%20this%20year.

174 *A rather magnificent piece of research called "Woman Count 2020"*: "Women-
Count2020 Role, Value, and Number of Female Executives in the FTSE 350," The
Pipeline, https://www.execpipeline.com/media/zitfa0aa/the-pipeline-women
-count-report-2020.pdf.

174 *According to the 2015 McKinsey Global Institute Report*: Lola Woetzel, Anu
Madgavkar, Kweilin Ellingrud, Eric Labaye, Sandrine Devillard, Eric Kutcher,
James Manyika, Richard Dobbs, and Mekala Krishnan, "The power of parity: How

advancing women's equality can add $12 trillion to global growth," McKinsey & Company, September 1, 2015, https://www.mckinsey.com/featured-insights /employment-and-growth/how-advancing-womens-equality-can-add-12-trillion -to-global-growth.

174 *151 years to close current gender gaps*: "Global Gender Gap Report, 2022," World Economic Forum, July 13, 2022, https://www.weforum.org/publications/global -gender-gap-report-2022/.

176 *In 2017, a 911 operator named Alisha Coleman*: *Coleman v. Bobby Dodd Inst., Inc.*, CASE NO.4:17-CV-29 (M.D. Ga. Jun. 8, 2017), https://casetext.com/case/coleman -v-bobby-dodd-inst-inc.

181 *The word "FemTech" was coined by Ida Tin*: Hannah Ward-Glenton, "Meet the woman who invented a whole new subsection of tech set to be worth $1 trillion," CNBC, March 8, 2023, https://www.cnbc.com/2023/03/06/meet-the-woman -who-invented-a-whole-new-subsection-of-tech-set-to-be-worth-1-trillion.html.

181 *There's Alloy Women's Health, which offers online menopause*: "The dawn of the Fem-Tech revolution," McKinsey & Company, February 14, 2022, https://www.mckinsey .com/industries/healthcare/our-insights/the-dawn-of-the-femtech-revolution.

182 *There are many companies paying lip service*: "Transcript: Mayor Eric Adams Delivers Address on Women's Health and Holds In-person Q-and A", January 17, 2023, https://www.nyc.gov/office-of-the-mayor/news/038-23/transcript-mayor-eric -adams-delivers-address-women-s-health-holds-in-person-q-and-a.

CHAPTER NINE: Pretty Menopausal

189 *But a 2014 component of SWAN looked at 405 women*: Kathryn L. Jackson, Imke Janssen, Bradley M. Appelhans, Rasa Kazlauskaite, Kelly Karavolos, Sheila A. Dugan, Elizabeth A. Avery, Karla J. Shipp-Johnson, Lynda H. Powell, and Howard M. Kravitz, *Archives of Women's Mental Health* 17, no. 3 (March 13, 2014): 177–87, https:// pubmed.ncbi.nlm.nih.gov/24623160/.

190 *Anorexia, bulimia, and binge-eating are by no means*: Danielle A. Gagne, BA; Ann Von Holl, MS; Kimberly A. Brownley, PhD; Cristin D. Runfola, PhD; Sara Hofmeier, MS, LPC; Kateland E. Branch, BS; Cynthia M. Bulik, PhD, "Eating disorder symptoms and weight and shape concerns in a large web-based convenience sample of women ages 50 and above: Results of the Gender and Body Image (GABI) study," *International Journal of Eating Disorders* 45, no. 7 (June 21, 2012): 832–44, https:// psycnet.apa.org/doi/10.1002/eat.22030.

190 *Furthermore, the highest rates of bulimia*: Paul Rohde, PhD; Eric Stice, PhD; Heather Shaw, PhD; Jeff M. Gau, MS; Olivia C. Ohls, BS, "Age effects in eating disorder baseline risk factors and prevention intervention effects," *International Journal of Eating Disorders* 50, no. 11 (August 31, 2017): 1273–80, https://doi.org/10.1002/eat.2 2775.

192 *There's a brilliantly observed passage*: India Knight, *Mutton* (London: Penguin Books Ltd, 2012), 10–11.

196 *As if all this wasn't enough, it's also been shown*: M. E. Levine, A. T. Lu, B. H. Chen,

D. G. Hernandez, A. B. Singleton, L. Ferrucci, S. Bandinelli, E. Salfati, J. E. Manson, A Quach, C. D. Kusters, D. Kuh, A. Wong, A. E. Teschendorff, M. Widschwendter, B. R. Ritz, D. Absher, T. L. Assimes, and S. Horvath, "Menopause accelerates biological aging," *Proceedings of the National Academy of Sciences of the United States of America* 113, no. 33 (March 18, 2016): 9327–32, https://pubmed.ncbi.nlm.nih .gov/27457926/.

201 *A 2017 study showed that MHT*: J. S. Passos-Soares, M. I. P. Vianna, I. S. Gomes-Filho, S. S. Cruz, M. L. Barreto, L. F. Adan, C. K. Rösing, S. C. Trindade, E. M. M. Cerqueira, and F. A. Scannapieco, "Association between osteoporosis treatment and severe periodontitis in postmenopausal women," *Menopause* 24, no. 7 (July 2017): 789–95,

202 *And hair can hugely affect mood*: "How it all started. Pantene and Yale University Reveals the Power of Hair," Pantene, https://www.pantene.co.uk/en-gb/power-of -hair/how-it-all-started/.

203 *It is said to affect up to forty percent of women*: Shannon Famenini, BS; Christa Slaught, BS; Lewei Duan, MS; and Carolyn Goh, MD, "Demographics of women with female pattern hair loss and the effectiveness of spironolactone therapy," *Journal of the American Academy of Dermatology* 73, no. 4 (October 2015): 705–706, https://www.ncbi.nlm.nih.gov/pmc/articles/PMC4573453/.

CHAPTER TEN: Hot Sex

211 *a digital issue entitled "Sex Life After 60"*: "Sex after 60, A *Special* DIGITAL ISSUE about the under-explored, under-discussed, under-celebrated sex experiences of experienced women," Cosmopolitan Digital Issue, 2024, https://www.cosmopolitan .com/interactive/a45893760/sex-after-60/#.

211 *it's depressing to see that its sister candle*: "Introducing: Hands Off My Vagina," Goop, January 20, 2022, https://goop.com/food/decorating-design/goop-hands -off-my-vagina-candle/.

218 *Buy the wrong product for your vagina or vulva*: S. E. Crann, S. Cunningham, A. Albert, D. M. Money, and K. C. O'Doherty, "Vaginal health and hygiene practices and product use in Canada: A national cross-sectional survey," *BMC Women's Health* 18, no. 52 (March 23, 2018), 10.1186/s12905-018-0543-y.

220 *sex does burn calories*: J. Frappier, I. Toupin, J. J. Levy, M. Aubertin-Leheudre, and A. D. Karelis, "Energy expenditure during sexual activity in young healthy couples," *PloS One* 8, no. 10 (October 24, 2013): e79342, https://doi.org/10.1371/journal .pone.0079342.

221 *Prolapse, where pelvic organs slip downwards*: L. Carroll, C. O. Sullivan, C. Doody, C. Perrotta, and B. M. Fullen, "Pelvic organ prolapse: Women's experiences of accessing care & recommendations for improvement," *BMC Women's Health* 23, no. 1 (December 18, 2023): 672, https://doi.org/10.1186/s12905-023-02832-z.

CHAPTER ELEVEN: Hormonious Relationships

227 *In a 2020 survey of fifteen hundred menopausal women*: Gill Shaffer, "Still a Taboo Subject?," Future You Cambridge, last updated May 2023, https://futureyouhealth.com/knowledge-centre/menopause-study-2020.

227 *Interestingly, in 2019, the aptly named MATE*: S. J. Parish, S. S. Faubion, M. Weinberg, B. Bernick, and S. Mirkin, "The MATE survey: Men's perceptions and attitudes towards menopause and their role in partners' menopausal transition," *Menopause* 26, no. 10 (October 2019): 1110–16, doi:10.1097/GME.0000000000001373. https://www.ncbi.nlm.nih.gov/pmc/articles/PMC6791510/.

229 *In 2017, an analysis of over two thousand adults*: Michael J. Rosenfeld, "Who wants the Breakup? Gender and Breakup in Heterosexual Couples," in *Social Networks and the Life Course: Integrating the Development of Human Lives and Social Relational Networks,* edited by Duane F. Alwin, Diane Felmlee, and Derek Kreager (Springer, 2018), 221–43.

230 *Rather sweetly, marriage hasn't lost its charm*: Christy Bieber, JD, "Revealing Divorce Statistics In 2024," *Forbes,* updated May 30, 2024, https://www.forbes.com/advisor/legal/divorce/divorce-statistics/.

230 *Interestingly, men are far more likely to remarry than women*: Krista K. Westrick-Payne, "Remarriage Rate 2021," Bowling Green State University, Family Profile November 19, 2023, https://www.bgsu.edu/ncfmr/resources/data/family-profiles/westrick-payne-remarriage-rate-2021-fp-23-19.html#:~:text=The%20remarriage%20rate%20has%20decreased,experienced%20a%20remarriage%20in%202021.

230 *Same sex marriages have been legal*: Catherine Schwartz, "What Percentage of Same-Sex Marriages End in Divorce?," Law Offices of Schwartz & Godbey, January 17, 2024, https://www.cschwartzlaw.com/2024/01/17/what-percentage-of-same-sex-marriages-end-divorce/.

233 *As we lose the hormones that exist to help us reproduce*: S. Maestrini, C. Mele, S. Mai et al., "Plasma Oxytocin Concentration in Pre- and Postmenopausal Women: Its Relationship with Obesity, Body Composition and Metabolic Variables," *Obes Facts* 11, no. 5 (October 30, 2018): 429–39, https://pubmed.ncbi.nlm.nih.gov/3037 2704/.

234 *I asked parenting expert Tanith Carey*: Tanith Carey and Dr. Carl Pickhardt, *What's My Teenager Thinking?* (DK, 2020).

234 *The median age to have a baby*: "Motherhood deferred: U.S. median age for giving birth hits 30," Associated Press, May 8, 2022, https://www.nbcnews.com/news/motherhood-deferred-us-median-age-giving-birth-hits-30-rcna27827.

236 *I found a study looking at women in recovery*: M. Guerrero, C. Longan, C. Cummings, J. Kassanits, A. Reilly, E. Stevens, and L. A. Jason, "Women's Friendships: A Basis for Individual-Level Resources and Their Connection to Power and Optimism," *The Humanistic Psychologist* 50, no. 3 (2022): 360–75, https://doi.org/10.1037/hum0000295.

CHAPTER TWELVE: Facing the Future

239 *In the award-winning show* Fleabag. Mary McNamara, "'Fleabag's' soliloquy on menopause is the best three minutes of TV ever," *LA Times*, May 24, 2016, https://www.latimes.com/entertainment/la-et-menopause-20190524-story.html.

239 *to an incredulous, martini-sipping Phoebe Waller-Bridge*: Phoebe Waller-Bridge, *Fleabag: The Scriptures* (Great Britain: Sceptre, 2019).

240 *I, for one shouted an* Hallelujah: Joshua Cohen, "Menopausal Drug Veozah Features Prominently Among Super Bowl Ads," *Forbes*, February 12, 2024, https://www.forbes.com/sites/joshuacohen/2024/02/12/menopausal-drug-veozah-features-prominently-among-superbowl-ads/?sh=59533b7e2.

240 *American feminist and suffragette Eliza Farnham*: J. Delaney, M. J. Lupton, E. Toth, *The Curse: A Cultural History of Menstruation* (Champaign: University of Illinois Press, 1988), 222.

241 *famed women's rights campaigner Marie Stopes*: Marie Stopes, *Change of Life* (London: Putnam, 1936), 135.

241 *Anthropologist Margaret Mead*: Helen D. Fisher, "Mighty Menopause," *New York Times*, October 21, 1992. https://timesmachine.nytimes.com/timesmachine/1992/10/21/809392.html?pageNumber=23.

241 *in 1963, the psychologist Bernice Neugarten*: Bernice L. Neugarten, Vivian Wood, Ruth J. Kraines, and Barbara Loomis, "Women's Attitudes Toward the Menopause," *Vita Humana* 6, no. 3 (1963): 140–51. http://www.jstor.org/stable/26761453.

241 *Michelle Obama talked about her own hot flashes*: Michele Obama, "What Your Mother Never Told You About Health," with Dr. Sharon Malone, *The Light Podcast*, September 30, 2020, 20:56, https://podcasts.apple.com/gb/podcast/what-your-mother-never-told-you-about-health-with-dr/id1532956108?i=1000493064968.

242 *In 2023, the magnificent Drew Barrymore memorably*: Carrie Wittmer, "Drew Barrymore Had Her First Hot Flash on Camera with Jennifer Aniston at Her Side," Glamour, March 29, 2023, https://www.glamour.com/story/drew-barrymore-had-her-first-hot-flash-on-camera-with-jennifer-aniston-at-her-side#:~:text=During%20the%20interview%2C%20Barrymore%20had,Whoa!%E2%80%9D.

242 *Oprah said of menopause*: "13 Celebrities Who Have Spoken Out About Menopause," *Glamour*, October 9, 2023, https://www.glamour.com/gallery/celebrities-who-have-spoken-out-about-menopause.

242 *Actor Gillian Anderson wrote a book*: Julie Mazziotta, "Gillian Anderson on Dealing with Early Menopause: 'I Felt Like Somebody Else Had Taken Over My Brain,'" *People*, March 13, 2017, https://people.com/health/gillian-anderson-perimenopause-depression/.

242 *Gwyneth Paltrow, who has endured ridicule*: Lauren Valenti, "Now Gwyneth Paltrow and Goop Want to 'Rebrand' Menopause," *Vogue*, November 2, 2018, https://www.vogue.com/article/gwyneth-paltrow-menopause-perimenopause-symptoms-hormones-mood-swings-sex-drive-goop-madame-ovary.

242 *Actor Tracee Ellis Ross has spoken*: Elizbeth Ayoola, "'I Can Feel My Body's Ability to Make a Child Draining Out of Me': Tracee Ellis Ross Gets Real About Perimeno-

pause," *Essence*, updated January 17, 2023, https://www.essence.com/lifestyle/tracee-ellis-ross-perimenopause/.

243 *According to a 2023 study involving over 460,000 participants*: S. Buecker, M. Luhmann, P. Haehner, J. L. Bühler, L.C. Dapp, E. C. Luciano, and U. Orth, "The development of subjective well-being across the life span: A meta-analytic review of longitudinal studies," *Psychological Bulletin* 149, nos. 7–8 (July–August 2023): 418–46, https://doi.org/10.1037/bul0000401.

243 *This phenomenon is explained in a study*: K. E. Campbell, L. Dennerstein, S. Finch, and C.E. Szoeke, "Impact of menopausal status on negative mood and depressive symptoms in a longitudinal sample spanning 20 years," *Menopause* 24, no. 5 (May 2017): 490–96. doi: 10.1097/GME.0000000000000805.

243 *postmenopausal women have a far more positive view*: L. Brown, V. Brown, F. Judd, and C. Bryant, "It's not as bad as you think: Menopausal representations are more positive in postmenopausal women," *Journal of Psychosomatic Obstetrics & Gynecology* 39, no. 4 (March 19, 2017): 281–88, https://pubmed.ncbi.nlm.nih.gov/28937311/#:~:text=Postmenopausal%20women%20held%20a%20significantly,05)%20women.

243 *Our confidence increases*: Jack Zenger and Joseph Folkman, "Research: Women Score Higher Than Men in Most Leadership Skills," *Harvard Business Review*, June 25, 2019, https://hbr.org/2019/06/research-women-score-higher-than-men-in-most-leadership-skills.

245 *As lifespan and working life extends*: "Changes in U.S. Family Finances from 2019 to 2022, Evidence from the Survey of Consumer Finances," October 2023, https://www.federalreserve.gov/publications/files/scf23.pdf.

245 *According to the AARP Longevity Economy Outlook reports*: The Longevity Economy® Outlook reports, a series of data analyses from AARP, https://www.aarp.org/research/topics/economics/info-2019/longevity-economy-outlook.html.

245 *As Forbes.com points out, women dominate*: Krystle M. Davis, "20 Facts and Figures to Know When Marketing to Women," *Forbes*, May 13, 2019, https://www.forbes.com/sites/forbescontentmarketing/2019/05/13/20-facts-and-figures-to-know-when-marketing-to-women/?sh=33aa3b3f1297.

246 *Only five to ten percent of marketing budgets*: Betsy Rella, "The undertapped power of the 50+ consumer," WARC, August 8, 2023, https://www.warc.com/newsandopinion/opinion/the-undertapped-power-of-the-50-consumer/en-gb/6284.

246 *In 2022, only ten percent of films featured a woman aged forty-five or older*: Dr. Stacy L. Smith, Dr. Katherine Pieper, and Sam Wheeler, "Inequality in 1,600 Popular Films: Examining Portrayals of Gender, Race/Ethnicity, LGBTQ+ & Disability from 2007 to 2022,", USC Annenberg Inclusion Initiative, August 2023, https://assets.uscannenberg.org/docs/aii-inequality-in-1600-popular-films-20230811.pdf.

246 *the 2024 Gender in Advertising Report by CreativeX*: Elissa Ha, Nicholas Wood, Isobel Bruce, Purvaja Patel, Collin Cummings, and Muniza Bridges, "Gender in Advertising 2024 Report," CreativeX, https://creativex.docsend.com/view/dkfxqb3cx7sixskz?__hstc=211672138.16f6f3a474a32c4e6f12de76a62806f1.1710621458542.1710621458542.1710621458542.1&__hssc=211672138.2.1710621458542&

__hsfp=2635398045&hsCtaTracking=63ec2f6a-b2fd-42e4-bc6b-5aadeef375
20%7Cc0112c8d 0c89 1c7c b12b 96od55533950.

248 *One brilliant science-led feature about skincare*: Kate Sandoval Box, "We Tried It: New Menopause Skincare for Estrogen Loss," Oprah Daily, April 5, 2023, https:// www.oprahdaily.com/beauty/skin-makeup/a43465953/menopause-skincare-for -estrogen-loss/.

248 *The global menomarket was estimated to be worth $17.8 billion in 2023*: "Menopause Market Size, Share, Growth Analysis, By Applications (Screening and Diagnosis), By End User (Hospital, Diagnostic Centres, Specialty Clinics, Others), By Region–Industry Forecast 2024–2031," Skyquest: Global Menopause Market, July 2024, https://www.skyquestt.com/report/menopause-market#:~:text=Global%20 Menopause%20Market%20was%20valued,of%20a%20woman's%20reproductive %20years.

249 *we also have the benefit of what's called crystallized intelligence*: Kendra Cherry, MSEd, "Fluid vs. Crystallized Intelligence: Balancing mental flexibility and accumulated wisdom," verywellmind, updated July 11, 2024, https://www.verywell mind.com/fluid-intelligence-vs-crystallized-intelligence-2795004.

249 *activities like reading tangibly increase intelligence*: Avni Bavishi, Martin D. Slade, and Becca R. Levy, "A chapter a day: Association of book reading with longevity," *Social Science & Medicine* 164 (September 2016): 44–48, https://www.science direct.com/science/article/abs/pii/S0277953616303689?via%3Dihub.

Recommended Reading and Resources

AHAH website: empowher.com/ahah

Blackgirlsguidetosurvivingmenopause.com

Bone Health and Osteoporosis Foundation: bonehealthandosteoporosis
.org

Daisynetwork.org

Faubion, Stephanie S., MD, MBA, *The New Rules of Menopause* (Mayo
Clinic Press, 2023)

Foxcroft, Louise, *Hot Flushes, Cold Science: A History of the Modern
Menopause* (Granta Books, 2009)

Haver, Mary Claire, *The New Menopause* (Rodale Books, 2024)

The Hot Years (subscribe via drmache.com)

Houck, Judith A., *Hot and Bothered: Women, Medicine, and Menopause in
Modern America* (Harvard University Press, 2006)

Madameovary.org (Dr. Mary Jane Minkin's website)

The Menopause Society, menopause.org

Index